616.3992 J677f
Johnson,
Fluids
demystified

W9-ADS-387

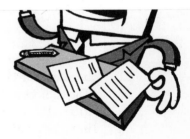

Fluids and Electrolytes Demystified

Notice

Medicine is an ever-changing science. As new research and clinical experience broaden our knowledge, changes in treatment and drug therapy are required. The authors and the publisher of this work have checked with sources believed to be reliable in their efforts to provide information that is complete and generally in accord with the standards accepted at the time of publication. However, in view of the possibility of human error or changes in medical sciences, neither the authors nor the publisher nor any other party who has been involved in the preparation or publication of this work warrants that the information contained herein is in every respect accurate or complete, and they disclaim all responsibility for any errors or omissions or for the results obtained from use of the information contained in this work. Readers are encouraged to confirm the information contained herein with other sources. For example and in particular, readers are advised to check the product information sheet included in the package of each drug they plan to administer to be certain that the information contained in this work is accurate and that changes have not been made in the recommended dose or in the contraindications for administration. This recommendation is of particular importance in connection with new or infrequently used drugs.

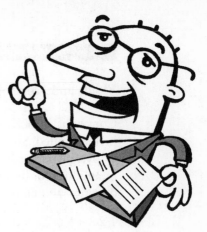

Fluids and Electrolytes Demystified

Joyce Y. Johnson, PhD, RN, CCRN

Dean and Professor, Department of Nursing
College of Sciences and Health Professions
Albany State University
Albany, Georgia

616.3992
J677f

With contributions by:

Edward Lyons, PhD

Professor of Biology, Department of Natural Sciences
Albany State University
Albany, Georgia

Bennita W. Vaughans, RN, MSN

Nurse Recruiter
Central Alabama Veterans Health Care System
Montgomery, Alabama

4/09

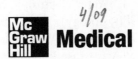 **Medical**

New York   Chicago   San Francisco   Lisbon   London
Madrid   Mexico City   Milan   New Delhi   San Juan
Seoul   Singapore   Sydney   Toronto

CUYAHOGA COMMUNITY COLLEGE
METROPOLITAN CAMPUS LIBRARY

The McGraw·Hill Companies

Fluids and Electrolytes Demystified

Copyright © 2008 by The McGraw-Hill Companies, Inc. All rights reserved. Printed in the United States of America. Except as permitted under the United States Copyright Act of 1976, no part of this publication may be reproduced or distributed in any form or by any means, or stored in a data base or retrieval system, without the prior written permission of the publisher.

1 2 3 4 5 6 7 8 9 0   FGR/FGR   0 9 8 7

ISBN   978-0-07-149624-7
MHID   0-07-149624-6

This book was set in Times Roman by International Typesetting and Composition.
The editors were Quincy McDonald and Robert Pancotti.
The production supervisor was Catherine Saggese.
Project management was provided by Tulika Mukherjee, International Typesetting and Composition.
The cover designer was Lance Lekander.
Cover design art directed by Margaret Webster-Shapiro.
Quebecor World, Fairfield was printer and binder.

This book is printed on acid-free paper.

Library of Congress Cataloging-in-Publication Data

Johnson, Joyce Young.
  Fluids and electrolytes demystified / Joyce Y. Johnson, with contributions by Edward Lyons, Bennita W. Vaughans.
      p. ; cm.
  Includes bibliographical references and index.
  ISBN-13: 978-0-07-149624-7 (pbk. : alk. paper)
  ISBN-10: 0-07-149624-6 (pbk. : alk. paper)
  1. Water-electrolyte imbalances.   2. Water-electrolyte balance
(Physiology)   I. Lyons, Edward, Ph. D.   II. Vaughans, Bennita W.   III. Title.
[DNLM: 1. Water-Electrolyte Balance.   2. Acid-Base Equilibrium.
3. Acid-Base Imbalance.   4. Body Fluids—physiology.
5. Water-Electrolyte Imbalance. QU 105 J66f 2008]
RC630.J64 2008
616.3'992—dc22

2007036095

To my mother, who has been my most powerful role model.
To my husband Larry, my daughter Virginia, and my son Larry, who love me unconditionally.
To my friends and family, who sustain me.
To my students, who provide my motivation to teach and to write.

ABOUT THE AUTHORS

Joyce Y. Johnson, PhD, RN, CCRN, serves as dean of the College of Sciences and Health Professions at Albany State University, with primary oversight for the undergraduate and graduate programs in the Department of Nursing and three additional departments. Dr. Johnson has been a nurse for over 30 years and a nurse educator for 25 years. She received her bachelor's of science in nursing from Vanderbilt University, her master's in nursing from Emory University, and her PhD from the University of Mississippi. Dr. Johnson is author of many nursing textbooks and book chapters, articles, and monographs. Her research areas are in curriculum trends in nursing programs and facilitating nursing student success, in addition to various clinical topics.

Edward Lyons, PhD, is a professor of biology in the Department of Natural Sciences at Albany State University in Albany, Georgia. Dr. Lyons has been a science educator for over 35 years and has taught biology and anatomy and physiology to many nursing students during his tenure. Dr. Lyons received his bachelor's and master's degrees from Howard University and his PhD in cell biology from Atlanta University.

Bennita W. Vaughans, RN, MSN, is a nurse recruiter at the Central Alabama Veterans Health Care System. She has been a nurse educator for over 20 years and has provided care to adults in many health care settings.

CONTENTS AT A GLANCE

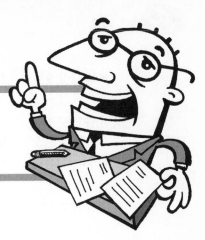

                and Hyperphosphatemia   135

CHAPTER 10   Acid–Base Imbalances   147

PART THREE   APPLICATIONS FOR FLUID AND
                ELECTROLYTE CONCEPTS

CHAPTER 11   Multisystem Conditions Related to Fluid,
                Electrolyte, and Acid–Base Imbalances   159

CHAPTER 12   Conditions Resulting in Fluid, Electrolyte,
                and Acid–Base Imbalances   185

                Answers to Final Check-ups   207

                References   211

                Index   213

CONTENTS

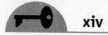

ACKNOWLEDGMENTS

Thank you to Quincy McDonald for providing this opportunity and for giving continuous positive energy to this project.

Thank you to Robert Pancotti for guidance through the preparation of the manuscript and for patience.

Thank you to Lynnette Johnson for assistance in manuscript preparation.

Thank you to Bennita Vaughans for her contributions to the manuscript.

Thank you to Dr. Edward Lyons for lending his expertise to the project.

INTRODUCTION

Fluids and Electrolytes Demystified is a detailed overview of the critical concepts involved in fluid, electrolyte, and acid–base balance and imbalance, collectively one of the hardest topics to master in undergraduate nursing. Fluid and electrolyte balance and acid–base balance have challenged students for ages. Some of the difficulty in understanding this content may lie in the attempt to remember each individual detail or symptom associated with an imbalance combined with the difficulty of mastering the physiology involved in each process. The list of symptoms of imbalance can be extensive; there is often duplication and overlap between electrolyte and acid–base imbalances. In *Fluids and Electrolytes Demystified*, the normal functions are discussed to provide baseline data. The concepts of imbalance are presented individually, but the links between concepts are addressed. The reader is led toward two facts: that many of the fluid, electrolyte, and acid–base imbalance symptoms are interrelated and that the imbalances themselves are interlinked.

Fluids and Electrolytes Demystified is a detailed, easy-to-understand overview of the concepts; it focuses on the information that students need most to understand the conditions that result in fluid and electrolyte imbalances. The book emphasizes the most critical information in fluids and electrolytes by discussing the underlying mechanisms involved in maintaining fluid, electrolyte, and acid–base balance and by discussing the factors that fail and result in an imbalance.

To promote understanding, there is coverage of the developmental changes and major conditions that result in fluid, electrolyte, or acid–base imbalances. The nursing assessments, interventions, and evaluations are reviewed to provide a whole picture of the patient's needs and nursing care situation. *Fluids and Electrolytes Demystified* contains clear language and helpful features to guide the student through application of concepts to real-life situations.

The content in *Fluids and Electrolytes Demystified* is organized as follows:

Chapters 1 and 2 are overview chapters that discuss the physiology involved in fluid, electrolyte, and acid–base balance. Chapter 3 discusses the diagnostic tests and basic nursing assessments related to fluid, electrolyte, and acid–base balance.

Chapter 4 focuses on fluid volume imbalances (i.e., hypervolemia and hypovolemia) and related symptoms and treatments. Chapters 5 through 9 present the major electrolytes and concepts related to excessive or insufficient blood levels of sodium, potassium, calcium, magnesium, and phosphate. Chapter 10 focuses on acid–base imbalances and discusses the procedures needed to determine the underlying source of the imbalance and the appropriate treatments and patient care needed to address the imbalance. Chapters 11 and 12 contain presentations of developmental conditions and disease conditions that involve imbalances in fluids, electrolytes, and acid–base, with the aim of enabling the reader to apply the concepts learned in earlier chapters of the book.

The reader is encouraged to review Chapters 1 and 2 to refresh his or her knowledge of the underlying processes involved in maintaining homeostasis through fluid, electrolyte, and acid–base balance. If the reader has a solid background in the physiology involved in these processes, Chapter 3 will be the best starting point. Once the reader has completed a thorough review of the material dealing with imbalances, the conditions presented in Chapters 11 and 12 should be explored to promote integration of knowledge from these chapters into actual patient situations.

The text features of *Fluids and Electrolytes Demystified* are organized as follows:

- Each detailed chapter begins with a list of Learning Objectives, each of which is discussed further in the text.

- Key terms are identified for the content area. These terms are **boldface** when first presented and defined in the chapter text to highlight them.

- A brief overview of the topic is provided.

- Content is divided into a brief review of normal function followed by detailed discussion of the imbalances that occur.

- Lists and bullet points are used to present key facts.

- Figures are provided to further illustrate concepts discussed in the text.

- Tables are provided to highlight and summarize important details.

- The "Speed Bumps" feature serves as a checkpoint that enables the reader to quickly gauge his or her understanding after a portion of the information is presented.

- A conclusion summarizes the content of the chapter.

- At the end of the chapter, a final check-up consists of NCLEX-style questions that test the reader's retention of the information from the chapter.

The reader is encouraged to become familiar with the key terms and their definitions because these are used throughout the book. If, at any point in the overview, the content seems unfamiliar, the reader should review the more detailed materials presented in the first two chapters of the book. The reader should examine the figures and tables to increase understanding and to view the interrelated nature of the content.

If the student cannot answer the questions asked in the "Speed Bumps" checkpoint, he or she should undertake a second review of the chapter or should review, at a minimum, the content covered in the question. Similarly, if the student has difficulty with a question asked in the final check-up section, he or she should review the entire chapter or related content.

Fluids and Electrolytes Demystified is not designed to be an exposure to the entire subject of fluids, electrolytes, and acid–base balance or imbalance. Thus the book does not discuss many cellular and biochemical functions related to total body mechanisms. For additional data, the reader is encouraged to consult a textbook on anatomy and physiology or on pathophysiology.

The content is presented in bulleted format whenever possible to allow direct focus on major points and on key aspects of the content. Although memorization is discouraged for most of the content in this book, and integration of concepts is essential for true learning, some facts presented in the bullet points, such as lists of foods containing certain electrolytes, must be memorized. When reading materials in a bulleted list, the reader should observe patterns or other similarities that will assist in remembering the items. For example, the symptoms of an imbalance may include memory lapse, confusion, and altered behavior, all of which are signs of altered neurostatus. The reader can associate the fact that the imbalance causes decreased conduction in neurons with the fact that such an imbalance can affect the nervous system and reasonably can result in changes in neurostatus.

To promote maximum learning, the reader should approach the material by looking for reasonable connections between altered physiologic function and symptoms that result from the alteration. Similarly, the reader should connect the assessments, diagnostic testing, and findings with the pathophysiology and possible symptoms associated with that pathology.

Fluids and Electrolytes Demystified is designed to make the concepts associated with fluid, electrolyte, and acid–base balance and imbalance clear and understandable. The key to demystifying the concepts is to see the connections and to make sense of the underlying processes involved, which will lead to an understanding of the imbalances that occur when normal processes fail.

Fluids and Electrolytes Demystified endeavors to illuminate the aspects of fluid, electrolyte, and acid–base balance that seem elusive and complex by breaking down the elements involved. The repetition of content from the overview chapters to the chapters dealing with imbalances is intentional to enable connections between the basic processes and the imbalances resulting from alterations in those processes. By understanding aspects of the processes involved in maintaining balance, one can more easily understand the imbalances that result when a process is altered or fails.

We believe that you will find *Fluids and Electrolytes Demystified* helpful in increasing your understanding of this difficult topic. As you move through course content and eventually prepare to take the nursing licensure exam (NCLEX), we hope that you will use *Fluids and Electrolytes Demystified* to promote successful completion and continued knowledge and understanding related to fluids, electrolytes, and acid–base balance and imbalances.

PART ONE

Foundational Concepts and Assessments

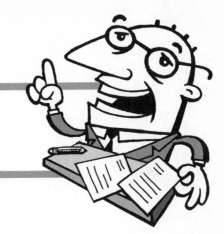

CHAPTER 1

Key Elements Underlying Fluid and Electrolyte Balance

Learning Objectives

At the end of this chapter, the student will be able to

1 Describe the process of fluid and substance movement into and out of the cell.

2 Contrast the regulatory mechanisms for maintaining fluid balance.

3 Distinguish between characteristics of fluid balance and fluid imbalance.

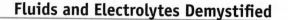

4 Contrast electrolyte balance and conditions of electrolyte imbalance.

5 Discuss the process for determining the effectiveness of a treatment regimen in restoring fluid and electrolyte balance.

Key Terms

Anions	Hypotonic
Cations	Hypovolemia
Diffusion	Interstitial
Electrolytes	Intracellular
Facilitative diffusion	Isotonic
Filtration	Osmolality
Extracellular	Osmosis
Homeostasis	Plasma
Hypertonic	Tonicity
Hypervolemia	

Overview

The human body is a miraculous machine. It functions, almost totally automatically, to produce energy and motion when supplied with essential fluid, nutrients, and oxygen. Through a delicate process of combining and breaking links between **cations** (positively charged molecules) and **anions** (negatively charged molecules), often referred to as **electrolytes,** chemical reactions are generated that release energy. This energy, in turn, results in mobility at the cellular level with active transport of electrolytes across membranes and tissue and organ mobility, such as a muscle fiber shortening and muscle contraction. This mobility proceeds to system activity, such as heartbeats that send blood throughout the body, and mobility of the entire body, such as in walking or running.

The most incredible mobility occurs at the cellular level when fluids and electrolytes are exchanged across membranes to maintain **homeostasis**, the balance in the body needed to sustain life. While some of these exchanges are passive and flow freely with little effort, other exchanges are active, energy-exhausting processes designed to maintain a critical balance of fluid and electrolytes on each side of the cell membrane and an environment that is appropriately charged with acids or bases to allow essential chemical reactions to occur. What is fluid balance? What are the electrolytes of life? This chapter will address these questions beginning with a basic overview of select anatomy and physiology of the human body.

The Cell

Cells are the basic unit of structure and function of life. Many organisms consist of just one single cell. This cell performs all the vital functions for that organism. On the other hand, many organisms are multicellular, including humans, whose bodies are composed of about 70 trillion cells in their own environment. Cells make up tissues, tissues form organs, and organs form organ systems, and these all interact in ways that keep this internal environment relatively constant despite an ever-changing outside environment. With very few exceptions, all body structures and functions work in ways that maintain life.

All cells are bounded by a plasma membrane. This membrane is selectively permeable—allowing certain things in and out while excluding others. Useful substances like oxygen and nutrients enter through the membrane, while waste products like carbon dioxide leave through it. These movements involve physical (passive) processes such as:

- **Osmosis**—water movement across a membrane from an area of low concentration to an area of high concentration

- **Diffusion**—movement of molecules from an area of high concentration to an area of low concentration

- **Facilitative diffusion**—movement of molecules from an area of high concentration to an area of low concentration using a carrier cell to accelerate diffusion

- **Filtration**—selective allowance or blockage of substances across a membrane, wherein movement is influenced by a pressure gradient

The movement of substances across a membrane also includes physiologic (or active) processes such as

- *Active transport*—molecules moving against a concentration gradient with the assistance of energy. Sodium and potassium differ greatly from the intracellular to the extracellular environment. To maintain the concentration difference, sodium and potassium move against the concentration gradient with the help of adenosine triphosphate (ATP), an energy source produced in the mitochondria of cells. This active transport process is referred to as the *sodium–potassium pump*. Calcium is also moved across the cell membrane through active transport.

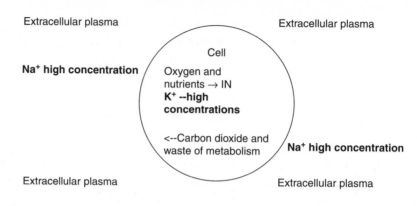

Extracellular plasma

Extracellular plasma

Na⁺ high concentration

Cell

Oxygen and
nutrients → IN
**K⁺ --high
concentrations**

<--Carbon dioxide and
waste of metabolism

Na⁺ high concentration

Extracellular plasma

Extracellular plasma

Figure 1–1   The relationship between the cell and its extracellular environment
regarding transport of electrolytes across the cell membrane.

- *Endocytosis*—plasma membrane surrounds the substance being transported
  and takes the substances into the cell with the assistance of ATP
- *Exocytosis*—manufactured substances are packaged in secretory vesicles
  that fuse with the plasma membrane and are released outside the cell

Figure 1–1 shows the relationship between the cell and its extracellular environment
regarding transport of electrolytes across the cell membrane.

Functionally, the membrane is active and living. Many metabolic activities take
place on its surface, and it contains receptors that allow it to communicate with
other cells and detect and respond to chemicals in its environment. Additionally, it
serves as a conduit between the cell and the extracellular fluids in the body's internal
environment, thereby helping to maintain homeostasis. If we are to understand
many aspects of physiology, it is important that we also understand the mechanism
by which substances cross the cell membrane. **1**

If cells are to survive and function normally, the fluid medium in which they live
must be in equilibrium. Fluid and electrolyte balance, therefore, implies constancy,
or homeostasis. This means that the amount and distribution of body fluids and
electrolytes are normal and constant. For homeostasis to be maintained, the water
and electrolytes that enter (input) the body must be relatively equal to the amount
that leaves (output). An imbalance of **osmolality,** the amount of force of solute per
volume of solvent (measured in miliosmoles per kilogram—mOsm/kg or mmol/
kg), of this medium can lead to serious disorders or even death. Fortunately, the
body maintains homeostasis through a number of self-regulating systems, which
include hormones, the nervous system, fluid–electrolyte balance, and acid–base
systems. **1**

Fluid

Water is a critical medium in the human body. The chemical reactions that fuel the body occur in the body fluids. Fluid is the major element in blood plasma that is used to transport nutrients, oxygen, and electrolytes throughout the body. Considering that the human body is composed of from 50 percent (adult females) to 60 percent (adult males) to 75 percent (infants) fluids, it is easy to understand that fluid must play an important role in maintaining life. Fluid intake should approximately equal fluid output each day to maintain an overall balance.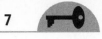

Intake of fluids and solid foods that contain water accounts for nearly 90 percent of fluid intake. Cellular metabolism, which results in the production of hydrogen and oxygen combinations (H_2O), accounts for the remaining 10 percent of water in the body (see Chapter 2). Fluid intake comes from the following sources (approximate percentages):

- Fluid intake (50 percent)
- Food intake (40 percent)
- Metabolism (10 percent)

Solid foods are actually high in fluid content, for example:

- Lean meats—70 percent fluid
- Fruits and vegetables—95 percent or more fluid

Excess fluid intake can result in overload for the heart and lungs and fluid deposits in tissues and extravascular spaces.

Fluid loss can occur from inadequate intake or from excessive loss from the body, most commonly from the kidneys. Fluid loss occurs from

- Urine (58 percent)
- Stool (7.5 percent)
- Insensible loss
  - Lungs (11.5 percent)
  - Skin—sweat and evaporation (23 percent)

Excess loss through perspiration and respiration or through vomiting or diarrhea may severely reduce circulating volume and present a threat to tissue perfusion. ◢3◣

Fluid is contained in the body in several compartments separated by semipermeable membranes. The major compartments are

- **Intracellular**—the area inside the cell membrane, containing 65 percent of body fluids

- **Extracellular**—the area in the body that is outside the cell, containing 35 percent of body fluids

  - Tissues or **interstitial** area—contains 25 percent of body fluids

  - Blood plasma and lymph—represents 8 percent of body fluids

    - Blood plasma is contained in the intravascular spaces

  - Transcellular fluid—includes all other fluids and represents 2 percent of body fluids (e.g., eye humors, spinal fluid, synovial fluid, and peritoneal, pericardial, pleural, and other fluids in the body)

Thus, most fluid is located inside the body cells (intracellular), with the next highest amount being located in the spaces and tissues outside the blood vessels (i.e., interstitial), and the smallest amount of fluid being located outside body cells in the fluid surrounding blood cells in the blood vessels (i.e., plasma).

Intracellular fluid balance is regulated primarily through the permeability of the cell membrane. Cell membranes are selectively permeable, allowing ions and small molecules to pass through while keeping larger molecules inside, such as proteins that are synthesized inside the cell. **1**

Some electrolyes are actively transported across the cell membrane to obtain a certain electric charge difference and a resulting reaction. Water moves across the cell membrane through the process of **osmosis,** flow from a lesser concentration of solutes to a greater concentration of solutes inside and outside the cell. If the extracellular (outside the cell) fluid has a high concentration of solutes, water will move from the cell out to the extracellular fluid, and conversely, if the concentration of solutes inside the cell is high, water will move into the cell. The ability of a solution to effect the flow of intracellular fluid is called **tonicity.**

- **Isotonic** fluids have the same concentration of solutes as cells, and thus no fluid is drawn out or moves into the cell.

- **Hypertonic** fluids have a higher concentration of solutes (hyperosmolality) than is found inside the cells, which causes fluid to flow out of the cells and into the extracellular spaces. This causes cells to shrink.

- **Hypotonic** fluids have a lower concentration of solutes (hypo-osmolality) than is found inside the cells, which causes fluid to flow into cells and out of the extracellular spaces. This causes cells to swell and possibly burst. **1**

Problems arise if insufficient water is present to maintain enough intracellular fluid for cells to function normally or if excessive water flows into a cell and causes a disruption in function and even cell rupture.

Extracellular fluid balance is maintained through closely regulated loss and retention to ensure that the total level of fluid in the body remains constant. Mechanisms are in place for regulation of water loss, such as secretion of antidiuretic hormone (ADH) to stimulation retention of water in urine, which helps to prevent excessive fluid elimination. The mechanism of thirst (also stimulated by ADH, as well as by blood pressure) is used to stimulate the ingestion of fluids and fluid-containing foods. **3**

Fluid regulation depends on the sensing of the **osmolality,** or solute concentration, of the blood. As more water is retained in the body solutions, the osmolality is decreased and can result in hypo-osmolar fluid that has a lower amount of solute than water. When water is lost from the body, the osmolality of body fluids increases and can result in hyperosmolar fluid that has a higher amount of solute than water. The body responds to an increase in osmolality by stimulating the release of ADH, which causes the retention of fluid and lowers the osmolality of body fluids.

Fluid exerts a pressure on membranes (i.e., hydrostatic pressure), and that pressure serves to drive fluid and some particles out through the membrane while others are held in. Solutes dissolved in fluid exert a pressure as well (i.e., oncotic pressure) that pulls fluid toward it. Inside the blood vessels in the arterial system, fluid level is high, and the hydrostatic pressure drives fluid out into the interstitial area (along with nutrients and oxygen). In the venous system, on the other hand, the hydrostatic pressure is low and the osmotic pressure is high because solute (including red blood cells and protein molecules) is concentrated; thus fluid is drawn into the veins along with carbon dioxide and metabolic waste (Figure 1–2). The pressure of the volume and solutes in the blood vessels provides blood pressure needed to circulate blood for perfusion to the tissues.

Fluid volume also plays a part in regulation of fluid levels in the body. Several mechanisms, in addition to ADH, respond to the sensation of low or high fluid volumes and osmolality. Neural mechanisms, through sensory receptors, sense low blood volume in the blood vessels and stimulate a sympathetic response resulting in constriction of the arterioles, which, in turn, result in a decrease in blood flow to

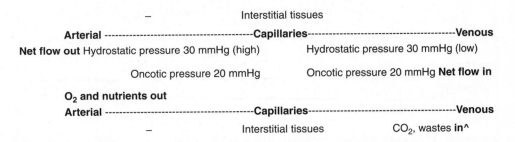

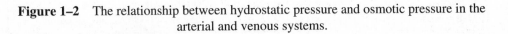

Figure 1–2   The relationship between hydrostatic pressure and osmotic pressure in the arterial and venous systems.

the kidneys and decreased urine output, which retains fluid. The opposite response occurs when high blood volume is noted.

- Arteriole dilation results in increased blood flow to the kidneys.
- This results in increased urine output and fluid elimination from the body.

The renin–angiotensin–aldosterone mechanism also responds to changes in fluid volume:

- If blood volume is low, a low blood pressure results.
- Cells in the kidneys stimulate the release of renin.
- This results in the conversion of angiotensinogen to angiotensin II.
- This stimulates sodium reabsorption and results in water reabsorption.

An additional mechanism for regulating sodium reabsorption is the atrial natriuretic peptide (ANP) mechanism:

- When an increase in fluid volume is noted in the atrium of the heart, ANP is secreted.
- This decreases the absorption of sodium.
- This results in sodium and water loss through urine.

When a decrease in volume is noted in the atria, ANP secretion is inhibited. Table 1–1 shows the relationship between fluid volume and renal perfusion.

Fluid volume regulation is necessary to maintain life. Decreased and inadequate fluid volume (i.e., hypovolemia) can result in decreased flow and perfusion to the tissues. Increased or excessive fluid volume (i.e., hypervolemia) can placed stress on the heart and cause dilutional electrolyte imbalance. It is clear that the renal system plays a vital role in fluid management. If the kidneys are not functioning fully, fluid excretion and retention will not occur appropriately in response to fluid adjustment needs. **2**

Table 1–1   Relationship Between Fluid Volume and Renal Perfusion

Low fluid volume → decreased renal perfusion	High fluid voume → increased renal perfusion
Stimulates	*Stimulates*
Renin–angiotensin–aldosterone release	ANP secretion
ADH secretion	Arteriole vasodilation
Sympathetic response → vasoconstriction	*Inhibits*
Inhibits	ADH secretion
ANP secretion	Renin–angiotensin–aldosterone secretion

SPEED BUMP

1. How does intracellular fluid regulation differ from extracellular fluid regulation?

    (a) Intracellular water balance is regulated through ADH secretion.

    · (b) Extracellular water balance is regulated through fluid volume and osmolality.

    (c) Intracellular water balance is regulated through aldosterone and renin secretion.

    (d) Extracellular water balance is regulated by fluid passage through cell membranes.

2. The body responds to low body fluid levels and increased osmolality with what actions?

    (a) Diarrhea

    (b) Diuresis

    (c) Tears

    ⁺(d) Thirst

3. Which mechanisms of fluid regulation respond to high fluid volume in the body?

    (a) Decreased ADH secretion

    ₀(b) Increased renin–angiotensin–aldosterone

    (c) Decreased water excretion

    (d) Increased sodium retention

Electrolytes

As stated earlier, *electrolytes* are electrically charged molecules or ions that are found inside and outside the cells of the body (intracellular or extracellular). These ions contribute to the concentration of body solutions and move between the intracellular and extracellular environments. Electrolytes are ingested in fluids and foods and are eliminated primarily through the kidneys, as well as through the liver, skin, and lungs. The regulation of electrolytes involves multiple body systems and is essential to maintaining homeostasis.

Electrolytes are measured in units called *milliequivalents* (mEq/L) per liter rather than in milligram weights because of their chemical properties as ions. The millequivalent measures the electrochemical activity in relation to 1 mg of hydrogen. Another measure that may be used is the millimole, an atomic weight of an electrolyte. This measure is often equal to the milliequivalent but on some occasions may be a fraction of the milliequivalent measure. Care should be taken when interpreting the value of an electrolyte to ensure that the correct measure is being used and that the normal range for that electrolyte in that measure is known. For example, 3 mEq of an electrolyte cannot be evaluated using a normal range of 3–5 mmol/L because you might misinterpret the finding. You must use the normal range in milliequivalents for proper interpretation. Table 1–2 shows the approximate ranges for electrolytes in both milliequivalents and millimoles. These values may vary slightly from laboratory to laboratory, so consult the normal values established at your health care facility.

The major cation in extracellular fluid is sodium (Na^+). Since sodium has a strong influence on osmotic pressure, it plays a major role in fluid regulation. As sodium is absorbed, water usually follows by osmosis. In fact, sodium levels are regulated more by fluid volume and the osmolality of body fluids than by the amount of sodium in the body. As stated earlier, ANH and aldosterone control fluid levels by directly influencing the reabsorption or excretion of sodium.

Another important cation is potassium (K^+). Potassium plays a critical role by influencing the resting membrane potential, which strongly affects cells that are electrically excitable, such as nerve and muscle cells. Increased or decreased levels

Table 1–2   Major Electrolytes, Their Functions, and Their Intracellular and Extracellular Concentrations

Major Ions	Function	Location	
		Intracellular	Extracellular
Sodium (Na^+)	Neuromuscular function and fluid management	12 mEq/L	145 mEq/L
Potassium (K^+)	Neuromuscular and cardiac function	150 mEq/L	4 mEq/L
Calcium (Ca^{2+})	Bone structure, neuromuscular function, and clotting	5 mEq/L	<1 mEq/L
Magnesium (Mg^{2+})	Active transport of Na^+ and K^+ and neuromuscular function	40 mEq/L	2 mEq/L
Chloride (Cl^-)	Osmolality and acid–base balance	103 mEq/L	4 mEq/L
Phosphate (HPO_4^-)	ATP formation and acid–base balance	4 mEq/L	75 mEq/L

of K^+ can cause depolarization or hyperpolarization of cells, resulting in hyperactivity or inactivity of tissues such as muscles. Potassium levels must be maintained within a narrow range to avoid the electrical disruptions that occur when the concentration of potassium is too high or too low. These disruptions can be life-threatening should they occur in vital organs such as the heart. Potassium levels are regulated primarily through reabsorption or secretion in the kidneys. Aldosterone plays an important part in control of potassium levels. If potassium levels are high, aldosterone is secreted, causing an increase in potassium secretion into the urine. **2**

Calcium (Ca^{2+}) is a third cation that is important to electrolyte balance. Similar to potassium, Ca^{2+} levels have an impact on electrically excitable tissues such as muscles and nerves. The level of calcium in the body is maintained within a narrow range. Low levels of calcium in the body cause an increase in plasma membrane permeability to Na^+, which results in nerve and muscle tissue generating spontaneous action potentials and hyperreactivity. Resulting symptoms include muscle spasms, confusion, and intestinal cramping. On the other hand, high levels of Ca^{2+} can prevent normal depolarization of nerve and muscle cells by decreasing membrane permeability to NA^+, resulting in decreased excitability with symptoms such as fatigue, weakness, and constipation. In addition, high levels of Ca^{2+} can result in deposits of calcium carbonate salts settling into the soft tissues of the body, causing tissue irritation and inflammation. Calcium is regulated through the bones, which contain nearly 99 percent of the total calcium in the body, as well as through absorption or excretion in the kidney and absorption through the gastrointestinal tract. Parathyroid hormone increases or reduces Ca^{2+} levels in response to the levels of Ca^{2+} in the extracellular fluid. Parathyroid hormone causes reabsorption of Ca^{2+} in the kidneys and release of Ca^{2+} from the bones and increases the active vitamin D in the body, resulting in increased absorption of Ca^{2+} in the gastrointestinal tract. Calcium and phosphate ions are linked, with high levels of phosphate causing low levels of available Ca^{2+}. Thus phosphate is often eliminated to increase available Ca^{2+} in the body. Calcitonin is another hormone that regulates calcium levels. Calcitonin reduces Ca^{2+} levels by causing bones to store more calcium. **2**

Magnesium (Mg^{2+}) is another cation found in the body. Like calcium, magnesium is stored primarily in the bones. Most of the remaining Mg^{2+} is located in intracellular fluid, with less than 1 percent being found in extracellular fluid. Magnesium affects the active transport of Na^+ and K^+ across cell membranes, which has an impact on muscle and nerve excitability. Of the small amount of magnesium in the body, half is bound to protein and inactive, and the other half is free. Magnesium levels are tightly regulated through reabsorption or loss in the kidneys. **2**

The major anion in extracellular fluid is chloride (Cl^-). Chloride is strongly attracted to cations such as sodium, potassium, and calcium, and thus the levels of Cl^- in the body are closely influenced by regulation of the cations in the extracellular fluid. **2**

Phosphorus, found in the body in the form of phosphate, is another anion in the body. Phosphate is found primarily in bones and teeth (85 percent) and is bound to calcium. Most of the remaining phosphate is found inside the cells. Phosphates often are bound to lipids, proteins, and carbohydrates and are major components of DNA, RNA, and ATP. Phosphates are important in the regulation of enzyme activity and act as buffers in acid–base balance. The most common form of phosphate ion is HPO_4^{2-}. Phosphate levels are regulated through reabsorption or loss in the kidneys. Parathyroid hormone decreases bone reabsorption of Ca^{2+}, releasing both Ca^{2+} and phosphate into the extracellular fluid. Parathyroid hormone causes phosphate loss through the kidneys, which leaves Ca^{2+} unbound and available. Low levels of phosphate can result in decreased enzyme activity and such symptoms as reduced metabolism, oxygen transport, white blood cell function, and blood clotting. High phosphate levels result in greater Ca^{2+} binding with phosphate and deposits of calcium phosphate in soft tissues.

Electrolytes are regulated through absorption and elimination to maintain desired levels for optimal body function. Just as indicated with fluid balance, although for some electrolytes not as detailed or formal in nature, electrolytes are regulated through feedback mechanisms (Figure 1–3). In some cases, as with sodium, the feedback mechanism involves hormone secretion (aldosterone) in response to serum osmolality and sodium levels. Similarly, in the case of calcium, parathyroid hormone and calcitonin are secreted to stimulate the storage or release of calcium from the bone to regulate levels in the blood. Other electrolytes are absorbed from foods to a lesser or higher degree or retained or excreted by the kidneys or bowels to a lesser or higher degree as needed to reduce or elevate the level of the electrolyte to the level needed for optimal body function.

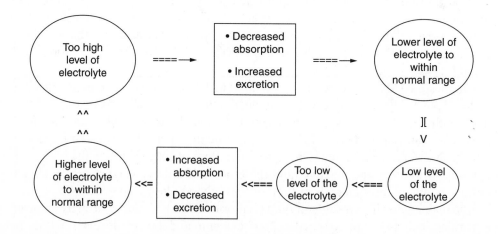

Figure 1–3   Example of feedback mechanism for regulation of electrolyte levels.

In order for the feedback mechanism to be effective, the organs or systems responsible for absorption and excretion (gastrointestinal) or reabsorption and excretion (renal) must function adequately. If the intestinal track is damaged or illness causes diarrhea or vomiting, absorption and excretion of electrolytes can be affected, and the feedback mechanism will malfunction. For example, in malabsorption syndrome, electrolytes are not absorbed through the tissue of the intestines to the degree needed, even though the levels of electrolytes are low.

Similarly, if renal system function is insufficient or nonexistent (failure), reabsorption and excretion of electrolytes may occur without response to the feedback mechanism or consideration of current levels of electrolytes. For example, in renal failure, potassium may be not be excreted and may even be reabsorbed, although the potassium level is already high because there is a failure of the usual feedback mechanism. Table 1–3 is a summary of regulation mechanisms for representative electrolytes.

Table 1–3   Regulation Mechanisms of Electrolytes

Electrolyte	Regulation Mechanism
Sodium (Na^+)	Aldosterone Antidiuretic hormone (ADH)—water regulation Atrial natriuretic peptide (ANP) Renal reabsorption Renal excretion
Potassium (K^+)	Intestinal absorption Aldosterone Glucocorticoids (lesser degree) Renal reabsorption Renal excretion
Calcium (Ca^{2+})	Parathyroid hormone Calcitonin Magnesium (helps in calcium metabolism and intestinal absorption) Intestinal absorption Renal reabsorption Renal excretion
Magnesium (Mg^{2+})	Intestinal absorption Renal reabsorption Renal excretion
Chloride (Cl^-)	Intestinal absorption Renal reabsorption Renal excretion

The regulation of electrolyte balance is important to maintain homeostasis. When regulatory mechanisms fail or are overwhelmed, electrolyte imbalances occur. It is important to be aware of the regulatory mechanisms and conditions that can affect the regulatory mechanisms to maintain electrolyte balance. ⬤5

SPEED BUMP

1. An imbalance of which cation is most likely to result in neuromuscular dysfunction?

(a) Sodium

(b) Potassium

(c) Calcium

(d) Magnesium

(e) All of the above

2. If a patient is experiencing symptoms of low calcium levels, would a decreased loss of phosphate owing to renal failure cause an increase or decrease in the symptoms?

Conclusion

Detailed discussions of the electrolytes will be presented in later chapters. Several key points should be noted from this overview chapter.

- The levels of fluids and electrolytes in the body have great impact on the body's ability to function effectively.

- The kidneys play a major role in regulation of the levels of fluids and electrolytes in the body. Thus anything that damages or inhibits the function of the kidneys affects the levels of fluids and electrolytes in the body.

- Several organs in the body produce hormones that affect fluid and electrolyte regulation, and removal or damage to one or more of those organs will affect the production of those hormones and thus the levels of fluids and electrolytes in the body.

- Electrolytes affect electrically charged cells, specifically nerves and muscles, with the potential for a critical impact on heart and brain function.

- Cations and anions are attracted to one another; thus the mechanisms that regulate cations will affect the regulation of anions.

- Bound ions are not active; thus removal of an anion can leave more unbound, available, and active cation in the body.

Final Check-up

1. Elise, age 5 years, has been vomiting for the past 4 days. She has been able to drink small sips of water but has vomited three times the volume she has taken in. She is admitted to the hospital with fluid and electrolyte imbalance. Which of the following is the nurse likely to observe?

    (a) Urine output of 100 mL/hour

    (b) Skin elastic and moist

    (c) Complaints of thirst

    (d) Dilute yellow urine output

2. If a patient is low on fluid volume, what reaction by the body would be the likely response?

    (a) High levels of ADH

    (b) Low levels of aldosterone

    (c) Low levels of renin

    (d) High levels of ANH

3. A high level of extracellular Na^+ will result in which of the following?

    (a) Low osmotic pressure

    (b) Low water level in extracellular fluid

    (c) High water retention in extracellular fluid

    (d) High movement of fluid from extracellular to intracellular spaces

4. Potassium is regulated through what mechanisms?

    (a) ADH causes a retention of potassium.

    (b) Renin–angiotensin causes an increased retention of potassium.

    (c) ANP causes an increase in potassium reabsortion.

    (d) Aldosterone causes potassium loss in the kidneys.

5. In what way is the available calcium level in the blood affected by phosphate levels?

    (a) High calcium levels will cause high loss of phosphate through the kidneys.

(b) High calcium levels will cause phosphate to bind with calcium, resulting in deposits.

(c) Low calcium levels will cause phosphate reabsorption and retention by the kidneys.

(d) Low calcium levels will stimulate a hunger for phosphate-containing foods.

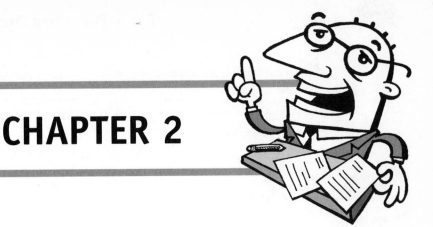

CHAPTER 2

Key Elements Underlying Acid–Base Balance

Learning Objectives

At the end of this chapter, the student will be able to

1. Explain acid–base balance.
2. Explain what is meant by pH.
3. Explain how hydrogen ions are expressed mathematically.
4. List the major sources of hydrogen ions in the body.

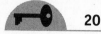
5 Distinguish between strong acids and weak acids and strong bases and weak bases.

6 Define buffer and explain how the buffer systems tend to restore changes in pH.

Key Terms

Alkalinic

Acidic

pH

Alkalosis

Acidosis

Buffer

Overview

1 Every metabolic reaction that takes place in the body is controlled by enzymes. Enzymes are biological catalysts that speed up and regulate chemical reactions without being consumed in the reaction. They are very specific and operate within very specific environmental conditions involving temperature and narrow ranges of pH, a gauge of acidity and alkalinity.

What Is pH?

2 The **pH** is a measure of the acidity and alkalinity of a solution. [H$^+$] represents the hydrogen ion concentration in moles (atomic weight in grams) per liter. The range of pH spans from **acidic** (numbers below 7.35) to **alkalinic** (levels above 7.5). The pH of a solution can be represented by the following formula:

$$pH = -\log_{10}[H^+]$$

This formula is the negative logarithm of the hydrogen ions present in 1 L of a solution. pH usually is expressed on a logarithmic scale (pH scale) because the range of possible values is very broad. Hydrogen ion concentrations are almost always less than 1 mol/L. **3** The logarithm of a number less than 1 is a negative number; therefore, a negative logarithm corresponds to a positive pH value. A solution with a hydrogen ion concentration of 0.1 g/L has a pH value of 1.0; a concentration of 0.01 g H$^+$/L has a pH of 2; 0.001 g H$^+$/L is a pH of 3; etc. The pH scale extends from 0 to 14, and each whole number represents a 10 fold difference in hydrogen ion concentration. For example, a pH of 4 has 10 times the hydrogen ion concentration as a pH of 5. Simply stated, the lower the pH level, the more acidic a solution is, and the higher the pH level, the more alkaline a solution is. It is important to note that solutions with pH higher than 14 and lower than 1 can be produced, but these do not occur under normal biological conditions.

Water molecules can ionize slightly to produce equal numbers of hydrogen ions (H$^+$) and hydroxide ions (OH$^-$). Pure water has a hydrogen ion concentration of 0.000,0001 (10^{-7}) mol/L. The logarithm is -7. The negative logarithm is 7; therefore, the pH is 7. Water, therefore, is a neutral solution because the number of hydrogen ions is equal to the number of hydroxyl ions. As the hydrogen ion concentration decreases, the pH number increases, and as the hydrogen ion concentration increases, the pH number decreases.

Acids

An *acid* is defined as any chemical that releases hydrogen ions (H$^+$) in solution. Since hydrogen is nothing more than a hydrogen nucleus or proton, acids are also called *proton donors*. When acids are placed in water, they release hydrogen ions (protons), which will cause the water to become more acidic (pH number decreases). The anion has very little effect on the acidity. Some acids are called *strong acids* (HCl) because they dissociate completely when placed in water. **4**

$$HCl \underset{}{\overset{water}{\rightleftharpoons}} \underset{proton}{H^+} + \underset{anion}{Cl^-}$$

Conversely, some acids are called weak acids because they only partially dissociate when placed in water. Carbonic acid (H$_2$CO$_3$) is an example of a weak acid. **5**

$$H_2CO_3 \underset{}{\overset{water}{\rightleftharpoons}} \underset{proton}{H^+} + \underset{bicarbonate\ ion}{HCO_3^-}$$

Hydrogen ions sources include various metabolic activities in the body. These activities produce **acidic** products such as

- Ketone bodies
- Phosphoric acid

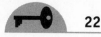

- Carbonic acid
- Lactic acid

These acidic products are constantly entering the body fluids, and they must be controlled. **4**

Bases

Bases are defined as proton or hydrogen ion acceptors. Most bases are chemicals that dissociate to produce hydroxide ions (OH^-). A substance that has a lower hydrogen ion concentration than hydroxide ion concentration is considered a base, so the addition of hydroxide ions to a solution makes the solution more basic. Since hydroxide ions (OH^-) act as a base and accept hydrogen ions (H^+), water is formed. Therefore, hydroxide ions tend to neutralize substances.

Like acids, bases can be either strong or weak. Strong bases dissociate completely, whereas weak bases dissociate only partially. Sodium hydroxide (NaOH) is a strong base and dissociates as follows:

$$NaOH \xrightleftharpoons{\text{water}} \underset{\text{anion}}{Na^+} + \underset{\text{hydroxide}}{OH^-}$$

Bicarbonate ion ($HCO3^-$) that forms from the dissociation of carbonic acid (H_2CO_3) acts as a weak base. Bicarbonate ion is a very important base in the body and is abundant in blood. **5**

SPEED BUMP

1. A solution that has an equal number of hydrogen (H^+) and hydroxide (OH^-) ions is called which of the following?

   (a) Strong acid

   (b) Strong base

   (c) Weak acid

   (d) Weak base

   (e) Water

2. If a patient is experiencing a physical condition that produces carbonic acid, what impact would ingestion of a bicarbonate of sodium have?

Acid and Base Balance

As stated earlier, the acidity or alkalinity of a substance is referred to as the **pH**. ⬤2 The normal pH of blood is between 7.35 and 7.45. High fever, taking too many antacids, or vomiting can cause the pH of blood to increase to above 7.46, a condition called **alkalosis**. If, on the other hand, the blood pH drops to below 7.34, then **acidosis** occurs. Acid–base balance is one of the most important aspects of homeostasis. The acid–base balance is concerned primarily with regulating the hydrogen ion concentration. The normal blood plasma pH range of 7.35–7.45 is maintained in the body when a 1:20 ratio of H_2CO_3 to HCO_3 is maintained.

⬤1 The optimal pH for enzyme function varies depending on where the enzyme is functioning in the body. For example, the enzymes that break down proteins in the digestive tract function at an acidic pH of 2, whereas those in the mouth that break down starches function at a pH of 7. Chemical reactions that take place in the extracellular fluids (ECFs) occur only when the pH is above 7. Deviations from normal pH actually can shut down metabolic pathways and lead to disastrous consequences.

Regulation

Changes in the pH of the body are resisted through varied **buffer** systems that convert a strong acid or base to a weak one and thus bind H^+ ions or leave more H^+ ions free. The body has several mechanisms for regulation of the acid–base balance of the body. The first mechanism is respiration. Respiration affects the acid–base balance by influencing the amount of carbon dioxide in the bloodstream. Carbon dioxide mixes with water to form carbonic acid, a weak acid, which breaks down into hydrogen ions (H^+) and bicarbonate ($HCO3^-$): ⬤6

$$H_2O + CO_2 \xrightleftharpoons{\text{water}} \underset{\text{Carbonic acid}}{H_2CO_3} > \underset{\text{hydrogen ion}}{H^+} + \underset{\text{bicarbonate}}{HCO_3^-}$$

This system is referred to as the *carbonic acid–bicarbonate buffer system,* and it regulates/buffers the blood pH by addressing high acid (H^+) levels in the blood by

- Removing CO_2 from the body (with deeper, more rapid breathing)
- Reabsorbing CO_2 in the kidneys and forming bicarbonate

This system functions best in an environment with a pH of 6.1 and would not be as effective outside the human body. The lungs and kidneys play critical roles in restoring order to pH management. Breathing out more CO_2 results in less CO_2 being available to bind with water to produce free hydrogen ions, thus resulting in less H^+ in the blood, and forming bicarbonate neutralizes acid by binding with H^+. Conversely, excessively low hydrogen ions in the blood would be buffered by retaining CO_2 in the body (through shallow, slower breathing) and by excreting CO_2 in the kidney and not forming bicarbonate, resulting in more free hydrogen ions and acid. Retention of CO_2 results in more CO_2 being available to bind with water to produce more free hydrogen ions, thus restoring the acid–base equilibrium of the blood. **6**

Respiratory control of pH is a rapid regulatory measure, occurring over minutes, but it has limitations and cannot be maintained as a long-term strategy for pH control. The limitations include the facts that (1) retention or release of CO_2 does not address the underlying cause of the imbalance, unless it is respiratory in nature, (2) extreme pH imbalances are not always fully corrected/compensated back to the normal level, (3) the energy needed for rapid breathing places a high demand on the body, and (4) decreased respiratory rate and depth can decrease oxygenation and compromise tissues.

The renal system is another major regulator of pH balance. The kidneys can control pH by secreting H^+ from the body or retaining it to reverse an acidosis or alkalosis. The renal mechanism can correct an acidosis by reabsorbing CO_2, which then combines with water to form carbonic acid and bicarbonate, which is released into the bloodstream, and H^+, as noted earlier in the carbonic acid–bicarbonate buffer system. The renal system can can correct alkalosis by excreting the CO_2, resulting in less bicarbonate formation.

In the renal buffering process, sodium (Na^+) is exchanged for hydrogen ions (H^+) and binds with some of the bicarbonate ($NaHCO_3$), which later breaks down again as Na^+ is actively removed through a Na^+–K^+ mechanism (discussed in more detail in Chapter 5). The H^+ ions are bound with carbonic anhydrase on the border of the proximal tubules of the kidneys, which convert the H^+ first to H_2CO_3 and then to H_2O and CO_2. Some H^+ ions also bind with the ammonia (NH_3) produced in the kidneys as a result of amino acid catabolism and an abundant anion found in the glomerular filtrate, chloride (Cl^-), to form ammonium chloride (NH_4Cl), a weak acid that is excreted in the urine. Thus it is clear that other electrolytes are involved in the acid–base balancing process and can be affected by acid–base imbalances. These impacts will be discussed with each electrolyte. **6**

Renal regulation of pH is a slow process occurring over a few days, but it can buffer large quantities of acid or base. Renal pH regulation results in a long-term, efficient correction of pH imbalance and, unlike the respiratory system, can fully return the pH to a normal range. Acute conditions cannot be corrected quickly by the renal system but over time can be well compensated by renal regulation. Respiratory conditions that result in acid–base imbalance can require renal regulation of pH and altered acid production, or base/bicarbonate production in the body (metabolic system) can require respiratory regulation of pH to restore acid–base balance. **6**

Another mechanism for regulating acids and bases in the body is the chemical buffer system. *Chemical buffers* are substances that combine with H^+ and remove it or release H^+ when it dissociates to allow more H^+ to roam free in the bloodstream. Two major chemical buffers are phosphate and protein. The phosphate system is a solution of HPO_4 and H_2PO_4:

$$H_2PO_4^- \rightleftharpoons HPO_4^{2-} + H^+$$

The most functional pH for this buffer system is 6.8, and this system works best in the renal tubules and intracellular fluid (ICF), where phosphates are more concentrated and the pH is optimal owing to constant production of metabolic acids, as opposed to the ECF, where bicarbonate is more readily available, and the pH is higher.

The protein buffer system is the most active chemical buffer system, handling three-quarters of the buffering of body fluids. The amino acid side groups associated with proteins bind with H^+ (NH_4) or release H^+ ($-COOH$) as indicated:

$$-NH_2 + H^+ = -NH_3^+ \quad \text{or} \quad -COOH = -COO^- + H^+$$

Proteins are more abundant than phosphate or bicarbonate and thus are an important chemical buffer system in the body. **6**

Conclusion

Detailed discussions of acid and base imbalances will be presented in later chapters. Several key points should be noted from this overview chapter.

- The degree of acidity or alkalinity in the body will affect the function of enzymes and metabolic activity in the body, thus affecting the body's ability to function effectively.

- The kidneys and lungs play major roles in regulation of the levels of acids and bases in the body; thus anything that damages or inhibits the function of the kidneys or lungs affects the acid–base balance in the body.

- Many electrolytes are affected by the body's attempt to regulate the H^+ ion level in the body; thus electrolyte imbalances can result from acid–base imbalance.

- The symptoms of acid–base imbalance may include exacerbated symptoms of electrolyte imbalance, most critically, neuromuscular and cardiac malfunction.

- Excessive mechanisms to correct an acidic condition can result in an alkalinic condition.

Final Check-up

1. Mr. Ellis, age 85 years, has been experiencing diarrhea for the past 4 days. He has been able to drink small sips of water but has had no other intake. The nurse suspects that an acid–base imbalance may occur and monitors for signs of the most likely imbalance. What symptom is the nurse likely to observe?

   (a) High blood pH

   (b) Low H^+ levels

   (c) Alkalosis

   (d) Acidosis

2. If a patient has breathing problems resulting in low blood oxygen levels and anaerobic metabolism, what state should the nurse monitor the patient for?

   (a) Low blood pH level

   (b) Alkalosis

   (c) Acidosis

   (d) Low hydrogen level

3. A person experiencing heartburn may take excessive bicarbonate of soda, resulting in what condition?

   (a) Low blood pH level

   (b) Alkalosis

   (c) Acidosis

   (d) High hydrogen level

4. If there is a high H^+ level in the blood, the body would attempt to balance it through what mechanisms?

   (a) Diuresis

   (b) Hypoventilation

(c) Hyperventilation

(d) Urinary retention

5. If the pH of the blood is below 7.30, what should the nurse monitor the patient for?

(a) Symptoms of the body's attempt to increase hydrogen ion retention

(b) Symptoms of the body's attempt to retain CO_2

(c) Symptoms of the body's attempt to decrease hydrogen ion retention

(d) Symptoms of the body's attempt to decrease bicarbonate

CHAPTER 3

General Nursing Assessments and Diagnostic Tests Related to Fluid, Electrolyte, and Acid–Base Balance

Learning Objectives

At the end of this chapter the student will be able to:

1. Distinguish laboratory values and assessment data that indicate fluid overload.

2. Distinguish laboratory values and assessment data that indicate mild to extreme dehydration.

3. Determine nursing assessments that are consistent with electrolyte imbalances.

4. Evaluate laboratory values and assessment data for indications of acid–base imbalance.

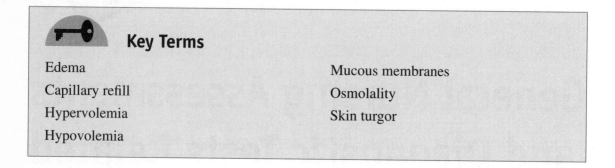

Key Terms

Edema

Capillary refill

Hypervolemia

Hypovolemia

Mucous membranes

Osmolality

Skin turgor

Overview

Laboratory testing is often used to confirm the presence and type of fluid, electrolyte, or acid–base imbalance the patient is experiencing. Nursing assessment often serves to confirm or contradict laboratory findings and facilitate the diagnosis and treatment of imbalances. Most diagnostic testing requires an order from the primary-care provider, but most nursing assessments, unless truly invasive, can be performed at the will of the nurse. Such assessments can be used to screen for possible imbalance or provide supporting data for diagnosis of a suspected imbalance and suggest the need for further, more invasive testing.

Laboratory testing involves collection of specimens, often blood and urine, and analysis of those specimens. Some testing can be done by the nurse, but most tests are performed in a laboratory setting. Timing can be critical for some tests. Some specimens are collected over a designated time period (24-hour urine tests). If blood or urine specimens are allowed to sit for hours prior to testing, the results can change and no longer be accurate (e.g., hemolysis of blood cells). It is important that the nurse secure an uncontaminated specimen and perform testing or delivery to the laboratory to perform the testing within as short a time frame as possible from the time of specimen collection.

Passing the Test

24-Hour Urine Test Procedure

- Best to start first thing in the morning.
- Urinate into toilet and record time.
- From this point on, void in urinal or specimen "hat."
- Pour urine from collection device into storage container provided.
- Continue to collect urine for entire 24-hour period (nights included).
- Do not add any more urine to the container beyond the time on the *next* day (i.e., start time 7 a.m. today, end time 7 a.m. tomorrow).
- Do not change your normal fluid and food intake.

Laboratory Test Units of Measure

Units of measure vary depending on the laboratory test being performed and the substance being measured. The basic units of measurement include the milligram (mg), which measures weight, and the liter (L) or deciliter (dL), which measures volume. A concentration of a solute (e.g., a medication) may be reported in milligrams per liter (mg/L). Electrolytes, however, are reported in units called *milliequivalents* (mEq). These units express the concentration of an electrolyte as a measure of chemical activity, not weight. The milliequivalent of an ion relates to its atomic weight divided by its valence (combining power of atoms measured by electrons it will give up, accept, or share).

Some countries use a measure called the *millimole* (mmol). The millimole is one-thousandth of a mole (the molecular atomic weight in milligrams). Many elements have the identical measures of millimoles and milliequivalents, but some elements are divalent (have a double valence) and will have a different millimole measure than milliequivalent measurement.

$$mEq/L = mmol/L \times valence$$

While a nurse would not be expected to calculate the millimole measure of an electrolyte, often the normal range of an electrolyte is expressed in both milliequivalent and millimole values. For some electrolytes, the nurse should be aware that the values are not the same and that the patient's level reported by the laboratory must be interpreted using the correct range for normal.

Solution concentrations may be reported in units measuring solutes per volume of water expressed in kilograms. These units are called *osmoles* (Osm). The osmolality, or tonicity, of a fluid is based on the number of osmoles or millisomoles per liter of water.

Laboratory Tests Indicating Fluid Imbalance

URINALYSIS: SPECIFIC GRAVITY

A principal laboratory test that indicates fluid deficit or excess is the urine specific gravity, which measures urine osmolarity. The normal range for specific gravity is 1.015–1.025. As fluid volume in the blood increases, the water excreted in the urine increases, making it more dilute and causing the specific gravity of the urine to decrease (below 1.015). Conversely, as the fluid volume in the blood decreases, as occurs in dehydration, the water excreted in the urine decreases, making it more concentrated and causing the specific gravity of the urine to increase (above 1.025). Some facilities have equipment on the unit that allows the nurse to perform a urine specific gravity test, but the urinalysis performed on admission and repeated periodically will include a specific gravity analysis. **1** **2**

HEMATOCRIT

Hematocrit levels also can indirectly indicate fluid volume in the blood. Since the test measures the number of blood cells per volume of blood, increased fluid in the blood, that is, **hypervolemia,** will dilute the blood cells and cause the hematocrit level to decrease. The normal range of values for men is 39 to 49 percent and for women is 35 to 45 percent. Consequently, too little fluid in the blood, that is, **hypovolemia,** will cause hemoconcentration and result in a high hematocrit level. It is therefore important to consider the patient's hydration level when interpreting laboratory values. For example, a hematocrit that falls within range or above range in a patient who is dehydrated actually may be low when the patient is fully hydrated. **1** **2** Use other laboratory values, such as specific gravity, to see a full picture.

SERUM OSMOLALITY

The test for **osmolality** measures the concentration of particles dissolved in blood. Sodium is a major contributor to osmolality in extracellular fluid. Serum osmolality generally ranges from 285 to 295 mOsm/kg of H_2O or 285 to 295 mmol/kg (SI units). As fluid volume decreases, as in dehydration, serum osmolality increases. Conversely, as fluid volume increases, as in fluid overload, serum osmolality decreases. **1 2**

URINE OSMOLALITY

The test for urine **osmolality** measures the concentration of particles dissolved in the urine. The test can show how well the kidneys are able to clear metabolic waste and excess electrolytes and concentrate urine. Urine osmolality, when the patient has maintained a 12- to 14-hour fluid restriction, has a normal level of greater than 850 mOsm/kg of H_2O or greater than 850 mmol/kg. In a random urine sample, the normal range is 50–1200 mOsm/kg of H_2O or 50–1200 mmol/kg.

Nursing Assessments for Fluid Imbalance

SKIN AND MUCOUS MEMBRANES

Skin turgor, or the time it takes for the skin to rebound once pinched together (particularly over the forehead in an elderly patient), can reveal the presence of dehydration. Slow rebound of skin, that is, poor skin turgor, is a sign of decreased tissue hydration, that is, dehydration. Skin also may feel dry to the touch if dehydration is present

    Edema, which is a swelling of tissues owing to the presence of excessive fluid, is noted when the patient is experiencing fluid overload or in some cases a fluid shift into tissues owing to trauma, such as a burn injury, or low protein levels in the blood, that is, decreased osmotic pressure (resulting in a fluid shift from hypo-osmotic blood to tissues—review colloid osmotic and hydrostatic pressure). Hypovolemia also will be manifested in patients by dry **mucous membranes** and possibly dry lips and tongue. Patients may complain of dry eyes capillary refill, which is the time required for blood to return to skin after pressure on the area (finger tips) causes pallor. Normal for capillary refill in 3 secs or less. Refill time 75 secs indicates decreased tissue hydration and perfusion. **1 2 3**

GASTROINTESTINAL AND URINARY

Constipation may be present with hypovolemia. Urine will appear concentrated with small volumes if hypovolemia is present. Urine will appear dilute or colorless with large volumes or urinary frequency (unless renal failure is present). **1 2 3**

Laboratory Tests Indicating Acid–Base Imbalance

The most common laboratory tests performed to determine acid–base status include an arterial blood-gas determination—pH, Pco_2, and HCO_3 levels, as well as Po_2 because hypoxia can result in lactic acidosis, venous serum CO_2, electrolytes because electrolyte levels are affected by acid or base states, and urine tests, including urinalysis, urine pH, and litmus dipstick tests.

ARTERIAL BLOOD GASES

pH

As stated in Chapter 1, the pH indicates the hydrogen ion concentration in the blood. There is an inverse relationship between the pH and the hydrogen ion concentration; thus an elevated pH indicates a decreased level of hydrogen ions, and a low pH indicates a high level of hydrogen ions. The normal range of the pH in the blood is 7.35–7.45 for adults and children. The pH range is slightly lower and higher for newborns and infants younger than 2 years of age, whose normal range of pH is 7.32–7.49.

The pH indicates an excess presence of hydrogen ions termed *acidosis* (pH < 7.35) or low levels of hydrogen ions termed *alkalosis* (pH > 7.45). The pH only determines the overall state of acid–base balance but does not indicate the source of the imbalance unless viewed in combination with other test values (Pco_2 and HCO_3).

Pco_2

The Pco_2 measures the partial pressure of CO_2 in the arterial blood and is an indication of ventilation. Commonly, 90 percent of the CO_2 in the body is in the red blood cells and 10 percent in the plasma. When a patient breaths, CO_2 is expired and removed from the body. The faster the respiratiory rate or the deeper the depth of respirations, the more CO_2 is expired. CO_2 is a metabolic waste product and contributes to the acid level in the blood. As the Pco_2 levels in the blood increase, the pH decreases, and vice versa. The normal range of Pco_2 is 35–45 mm Hg for adults and 26–41 mm Hg for children younger than 2 years of age.

HCO_3/Bicarbonate

Most of the CO_2 in the body is combined in the form of HCO_3. Bicarbonate is a weak base and represents metabolic waste in the body. The level of HCO_3 is regulated by renal excretion or reabsorption as needed to regulate acid–base balance. Bicarbonate has a direct relationship with pH. As bicarbonate levels increase, the pH level increases. The normal range of HCO_3 is 21–45 mEq/L for adults and 16–24 mEq/L for newborns and infants.

Po_2

The Po_2 is an indirect measure of oxygen content in the arterial blood. It measures the tension of O_2 dissolved in the plasma. The normal range is 80–100 mm Hg for adults and 60–70 mm Hg for newborns. The Po_2 level indicates how effective ventilation is in providing oxygen for the tissues. Oxygen levels can be affected by any condition that blocks oxygen delivery to the lungs or across the lung tissue into the blood. If oxygen levels are too low, metabolism must occur in an environment without oxygen (i.e., anaerobic) and produces lactic acid, which contributes to metabolic acidosis. 4

Base Excess

Base excess is a calculated value representing the amount of buffering anions in the blood (primarily HCO_3 but also hemoglobin, proteins, phosphates, and others). The normal range of base excess is ± 2 mEq/L. A negative base excess (–3 mEq/L or less) indicates a deficit of base and a metabolic acidosis (i.e., ketoacidosis or lactic acidosis). A positive base excess (3 mEq/L or more) indicates metabolic alkalosis (may be present in compensation for a respiratory acidosis). 4

ADDITIONAL BLOOD MEASURES

CO_2

The CO_2 content is an indirect measure of bicarbonate in the blood. Since most of the CO_2 in the body is in the form of HCO_3, the CO_2 content indicates the status of base in the body. The venous CO_2 level is commonly included when routine electrolyte levels are measured and should not be confused with the Pco_2 that is found in arterial blood and measures respiratory acid. The normal range for CO_2 content is 23–30 mEq/L (or mmol/L) for adults, 20–28 mEq/L (or mmol/L) for infants and children, and 13–22 mEq/L (or mmol/L) for newborns. The CO_2 level, as an indication of the bicarbonate level, is regulated by the kidneys. An elevated CO_2 level indicates metabolic alkalosis, whereas a decreased CO_2 level indicates metabolic acidosis. 4

O$_2$ Saturation

Oxygen (O$_2$) saturation is a measure of the percentage of hemoglobin (Hbg) saturated with oxygen. Oxygen bound to the iron in hemoglobin is referred to as *oxyhemoglobin*. The normal range is 92 to 100 percent, which is the level at which tissues will be oxygenated adequately if normal hemoglobin *dissociation* (i.e., oxygen separation from hemoglobin to move to the tissues) occurs. At oxygen saturation levels that are less than 70 percent, tissues are unable to extract enough oxygen from the hemoglobin to function properly. **◀4**

The oxyhemoglobin dissociation curve represents the increase in tissue oxygenation at higher hemoglobin saturation levels that occur under normal circumstances. It is not critical to dissect the oxyhemoglobin dissociation curve, but it is important to understand the principles represented; that is, as oxyhemoglobin increases, tissue oxygenation increases relatively proportionately. Circumstances can cause a decrease in hemoglobin's affinity (i.e., attraction) for oxygen and will help tissues to extract oxygen from hemoglobin and thus receive adequate oxygen at lower O$_2$ saturation levels. Conversely, certain circumstances will cause an increase in hemoglobin's affinity for oxygen, decreasing dissociation and causing tissues to be unable to extract oxygen from hemoglobin even if oxygen saturation levels are within an acceptable range (Table 3–1).

Basically, as cellular metabolism occurs, temperatures increase at the tissue level, waste builds up, CO$_2$ levels increase, and the pH decreases. Under these circumstances, the need for oxygen is high; thus the decrease in hemoglobin's affinity for oxygen provides more oxygen for the tissues at a time when the tissues

Table 3–1   Relationship Between Oxyhemoglobin Dissociation and Hemoglobin
Affinity for Oxygen

Conditions Causing Increased Oxyhemoglobin Dissociation and Tissue Oxygenation Owing to Decreased Hemoglobin Affinity for Oxygen	Conditions Causing Decreased Oxyhemoglobin Dissociation and Tissue Oxygenation Owing to Decreased Hemoglobin Affinity for Oxygen
Decreased pH (acidosis)	Increased pH (alkalosis)
CO$_2$ accumulation	Low CO$_2$ levels
Increased 2,3-diphosphoglycerate (2,3-DPG), a substance produced in RBCs when oxygen is low in the blood	Decreased 2,3-diphosphoglycerate (2,3-DPG), a substance produced in red blood cells (RBCs) when oxygen is low in the blood
Temperature elevation (hyperthermia)	Temperature decrease (hypothermia)
	Carbon monoxide (binds with hemoglobin and blocks oxygen binding)

need it. When the need is not as great, hemoglobin's affinity is increased, and oxygen is attached more quickly in the lungs and released less easily at the tissue level.

Oxygen saturation is calculated in the blood-gas equipment but involves the following formula:

$$\text{Percent of oxygen saturation} = \text{volume of } O_2 \text{ content Hbg} / \text{volume of } O_2 \text{ Hbg capacity}$$

Oxygen saturation levels can be determined through a noninvasive method called *pulse oximetry*. The pulse oximetry sensor can be attached to a fingernail or earlobe or any body surface on which it can transmit light from one side and record the light returned on the other side and calculate oxygen saturation. *Note:* Pulse oximetry records any oxygen-saturated hemoglobin and also will read *carboxyhemoglobin* (a deadly substance resulting from smoke inhalation or some inhalants). The nurse must note the patient's history to determine if a false elevation of the oxygen saturation level is present owing to carboxyhemoglobin. Assessment of the patient is vital to note if respiratory distress is present even though the oxygen saturation level is within normal limits. **3** **4**

O$_2$ Content

The O_2 content is a calculated measure of the amount of oxygen in the blood and will vary from arterial to venous blood. The normal range of venous O_2 content is 11–16 vol%, and the normal range in the arterial system is 15–22 vol%. Most oxygen in the blood is bound to hemoglobin and is referred to as *oxyhemoglobin*. The formula for O_2 content is

$$O_2 \text{ content} = O_2 \text{ saturation} \times \text{Hbg} \times 1.34 + \text{Po}_2 \times 0.003$$

O_2 content indicates the effectiveness of respiratory effort and ventilation. However, as the formula indicates, the amount of hemoglobin present in the blood, in addition to the effectiveness of ventilation, will affect the level of oxygen content. If the O_2 content is elevated, it indicates adequate ventilation and oxygenation of the blood. If the O_2 content is decreased, it may indicate inadequate ventilation (i.e., pulmonary disease) or decreased hemoglobin (e.g., as in anemia). **4**

Hemoglobin

The hemoglobin test is a measure of the total hemoglobin in the blood and indirectly indicates the RBC count. The test usually is done with the complete blood test. Decreased levels indicate the presence of anemia, that is, a low RBC count. Hemoglobin is composed of heme (iron surrounded by protoporphyrin) and globin (consisting of an alpha and a beta polypeptide chain). The iron in hemoglobin attracts oxygen, which makes it the perfect vehicle to transport oxygen to the tissues.

Normal ranges for hemoglobin, which may be slightly lower for the elderly, are as follows:

- Male adult: 14–18 g/dL or 87–11.2 mmol/L
- Female adult: 12–16 g/dL or 7.4-9.9 mmol/L (pregnancy > 11 g/dL)
- Child/adolescent:
  - Newborn: 14–24 g/dL
  - 0–2 weeks: 12–20 g/dL
  - 3–6 months: 10–17 g/dL
  - 6 months–6 years: 9.5–14 g/dL
  - 6–18 years: 10–15.5 g/dL

Deficient hemoglobin levels are problematic because of the strain placed on the cardiopulmonary system by the lower oxygen-carrying capacity. The heart rate and respiratory rate are elevated to provide adequate oxygen by circulating the limited blood cells as quickly as possible and providing as much oxygen to the blood cells as possible. If hypoxemia results from the low hemoglobin level, anaerobic metabolism and lactic acidosis could occur.

Excessive hemoglobin usually is present with a high RBCl count. High hemoglobin levels could result in problems owing to viscous (i.e., thick) blood with clot formation and resulting obstruction of blood vessels leading to ischemia and tissue death (e.g., stroke, angina, and heart attack).

Acid–Base Balance Assessment

STEPS IN BLOOD-GAS ANALYSIS

1. Note the pH and determine if the patient has an overall alkalosis (pH > 7.45) or acidosis (pH < 7.35).
2. Look at the P_{CO_2} level to determine if
   a. The P_{CO_2} level matches (is inverse to) the overall state (i.e., the pH is elevated [alkalosis] and the P_{CO_2} is decreased [alkalosis] or the patient's pH is decreased [acidosis] and the P_{CO_2} is elevated [acidosis]).

    b. If yes, then the state is due to the respiratory system and is a respiratory alkalosis or acidosis.

    c. If no match is noted (i.e., the pH indicates alkalosis, whereas the P_{CO_2} is higher than normal range [acidosis]), the respiratory system is not the cause of the imbalance, but it could be above or below normal to buffer a metabolic imbalance.

    d. Evaluate the base excess to determine if the acidosis or alkalosis is metabolic in nature.

3. Look at the HCO_3 level to determine if

    a. The HCO_3 level matches (direct relationship) the overall state (i.e., pH is elevated [alkalosis] and the HCO_3 is elevated [alkalosis] or the patient's pH is decreased [acidosis] and the P_{HCO_3} is decreased [acidosis]).

    b. If yes, then the state is due to the metabolic system and is a metabolic alkalosis or respiratory acidosis.

    c. If no match is noted (i.e., the pH indicates alkalosis, whereas the HCO_3 is lower than normal [acidosis]), the imbalance is not metabolic in origin, but the bicarbonate could be above or below normal to buffer a chronic respiratory imbalance.

    d. Evaluate the base excess to determine if the acidosis or alkalosis is metabolic in nature.

ALKALOSIS

- Blood gases show a pH > 7.45.
- Tests for pH will indicate alkalosis by color change on litmus paper or dipstick test.
- If the basis for the alkalosis is respiratory, the tests for CO_2 would indicate a decreased level, with the $Paco_2$ less than 35 mm Hg (6 kPa).
- If the basis for the alkalosis is metabolic, an elevated level of HCO_3/bicarbonate at 29 mEq/L or above would be noted.
- Metabolic alkalosis also might reveal an elevated serum CO_2 content (30 mEq/L or higher) as an indirect measure of bicarbonate.
- Metabolic alkalosis will reveal a positive base excess.

🔑 Nursing Assessments for Alkalosis

The nurse should monitor patients who are at risk for respiratory alkalosis closely, including those with

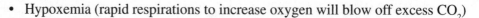

- Hypoxemia (rapid respirations to increase oxygen will blow off excess CO_2)
- Carbon monoxide poisoning (results in hypoxemia and hyperventilation with excess CO_2 loss)
- Pulmonary emboli (rapid respirations to increase oxygen will blow off excess CO_2)
- Anxiety (hyperventilation)
- Pain
- Pregnancy

The nurse also should monitor patients at risk for metabolic alkalosis closely, including those with or at risk for

- Hypokalemia (secondary to diuretic use or other potassium loss, which moves hydrogen ion into the cell)
- Hypochloremia
- Gastric suction
- Chronic vomiting
- Aldosteronism (decreases potassium)
- Severe diarrhea
- Hypoxemia resulting in anaerobic metabolism and lactic acidosis

The nurse may note such symptoms as

- Neurologic symptoms ranging from light-headedness to confusion, stupor, or coma
- Muscle twitching or hand tremor
- Muscle spasms (tetany) owing to calcium changes
- Numbness or tingling in the face or extremities
- Nausea and/or vomiting

ACIDOSIS

- Blood gases show pH < 7.35.
- In respiratory acidosis, $Paco_2$ will be high (> 45 mm Hg, or 6 kPa).
- Tests for pH will indicate alkalosis by color change on litmus paper or dipstick test.
- Respiratory acidosis that is chronic may reveal a positive base excess owing to an attempt to buffer the respiratory acid.

- Metabolic acidosis will reveal an HCO_3/bicarbonate level of 20 mEq/L or lower.
- Metabolic acidosis also will reveal a serum CO_2 content of 23 mEq/L or lower.
- Metabolic acidosis will reveal a negative base excess (–3 mEq/L or lower).

Nursing Assessments for Acidosis

The nurse should monitor patients who are at risk for respiratory acidosis closely, including those with

- Pulmonary disease
- Head trauma
- Oversedation resulting in decreased ventilation

The nurse also should monitor patients at risk for metabolic acidosis closely, including those with or at risk for

- Diabetic ketoacidosis
- Shock
- Renal failure
- Chronic use of loop diuretics
- Intestinal fistula
- Severe diarrhea
- Hypoxemia resulting in anaerobic metabolism and lactic acidosis

The nurse also must observe for symptoms related to the acidotic state, including

- Neurochanges such as coma
- Respiratory compensation with hyperventilation
- Deep Kussmaul breathing
- Respiratory exhaustion leading to respiratory failure

SPEED BUMP

1. *The nurse suspects that Mr. Brown is dehydrated. To confirm this suspicion, the nurse might expect Mr. Brown's assessment to show what findings?*

   (a) A decreased hematocrit level

   (b) An increased urine specific gravity

   (c) Moist mucous membranes

   (d) Decreased skin turgor rebound

2. *Which laboratory test results would support the diagnosis of fluid volume excess?*

    (a) Specific gravity of 1.005

    (b) Specific gravity of 1.020

    (c) Specific gravity of 1.030

    (d) Specific gravity of 1.036

3. *The patient with a chronic respiratory condition resulting in poor ventilation might demonstrate what diagnostic findings?*

    (a) pH of 7.45 or higher

    (b) P_{CO_2} of 35 mm Hg or lower

    (c) HCO_3 of 22 mEq/L or lower

    (d) P_{O_2} of 80 mm Hg or higher

Laboratory Tests Indicating Electrolyte Imbalance

Most facilities have on-site laboratories or will collect blood and body fluids to send to an outside laboratory. Electrolytes are measured directly by evaluation of blood levels or some through urine levels to determine the degree of excretion. Serum (blood) electrolytes may reveal a low (hypo) or elevated (hyper) electrolyte state. The common electrolytes measured in patients are potassium, sodium, and chloride, and additional test may be done to assess calcium, phosphate, and magnesium. Normal ranges for electrolytes may differ depending on the patient's gender, age, size, or or ethnic background and also may vary slightly from one facility or laboratory to another. Generally, the normal ranges for electrolytes are

- Potassium (K^+): 3.5–5.0 mEq/L, or in SI units, 3.5–5.0 mmol/L

- Sodium (Na^+): 135–145 mEq/L, or 135–145 mmol/L

- Chloride (Cl^-): 98–106 mEq/L, or 98–108 mmol/L

- Calcium (Ca^{2+}), serum: 8.5–10.5 mg/dL, or 2.1–2.7 mmol/L, for adults; can elevate to 12 mg/dL in childen with growth spurts and bone growth

- Calcium, urine: 0–300 mg/24 h, or 0.0–7.5 mmol/24 h. Ionized calcium (serum calcium not bound to protein) ranges in adults from 4.65 to 5.28 mg/dL. The level of ionized calcium in the blood is not affected by the amount of protein in the blood.

- Magnesium (Mg^{2+}): 1.3–2.1 mEq/L (1.4–1.7 mEq/L in children), or 0.65–1.05 mmol/L

- Phosphate ($HPO4^-$): 3.0–4.5 mg/dL (4–6.5 mg/dL in children), or 0.97–1.45 mmol/L (1.45–2.1 mmol/L in children). Values in the elderly may be lower than adult values, and newborns may have higher values than children.

Nursing Assessments for Electrolyte Imbalance

Knowledge of the common causes of electrolyte imbalances indicates the patient who is at risk and who should be observed most closely for signs of an electrolyte imbalance. Many symptoms and observations may result from one or a combination of electrolyte imbalances. Some symptoms are common to both hypo and hyper states of an electrolyte. Symptoms noted may indicate a need for laboratory testing to determine the exact imbalance and provide additional data to support the diagnosis. 3

Potassium

Potassium is the major cation inside the cell. Intracellular potassium accounts for 98 percent of the potassium in the body, whereas the remaining 2 percent is found in extracellular fluid. Potassium is critical to neuromuscular function because it plays an important role in action potentials, nerve polarization/depolarization, and excitability.

Some drugs may cause an increase or decrease in potassium levels and should be noted when levels are analyzed. Diuretics may reduce potassium (i.e., may cause an initial increase followed by diuresis and an ultimate decrease). The list is extensive but includes

- Aspirin (acetylsalicylic acid or other salicylates)
- Amphotericin B
- Bicarbonate (alkalosis)

- Intravenous (IV) theophylline
- Digoxin
- Diuretics (furosemide)
- Hydrocortisone
- Isoniazide
- Lithium
- Enalapril
- Bisacodyl
- Albuterol

HYPOKALEMIA

Low serum potassium, below 3.4 mEq/L (3.4 mmol/L), may be caused by the use of diuretic medications that result in the excretion of potassium in the urine and by the loss of potassium through diarrhea or excessive sweating. Deficient dietary intake of potassium and magnesium (which causes potassium to move into the cells) could contribute to the development of hypokalemia.

Symptoms the nurse may notice include

- Irregular heart rhythm and cardiac dysrhythmia (use a defibrillator for a quick check of heart rhythm if an electrocardiogram [ECG] has not been ordered and telemetry monitor is not available)
- General discomfort or irritability
- Muscle weakness
- Paralysis
- Hyperglycemia (check glucose levels; hypokalemia can cause decreased insulin release and decreased sensitivity to insulin)
- Rhabdomyolysis (i.e., disintegration of muscle fibers with myoglobinuria owing to hypokalemia, which can reduce blood flow to skeletal muscles)
- Renal impairment owing to prolonged hypokalemia with dilute urine (inability to concentrate urine), polyuria, nocturia, and polydipsia

3 Symptoms of hypokalemia may indicate the need for a urinalysis and blood tests to determine the amount of potassium being excreted by the kidneys and related electrolyte and acid–base imbalances.

HYPERKALEMIA

Hyperkalemia is excessively elevated potassium levels, that is, higher than 5.1 mEq/L (5.1 mmol/L), and it results most commonly from decreased excretion of potassium owing to renal failure but also may result from excessive intake or overaggressive treatment of potassium deficit with potassium supplements. In addition, deficient aldosterone levels, that is, Addison's disease, or aldosterone-inhibiting diuretics may cause hyperkalemia. Acidosis also can cause hyperkalemia by causing a shift of hydrogen ions into the cell and potassium ions out of the cell and into the blood. Transfusion of hemolyzed blood also can result in high potassium levels. Leukemic patients may demonstrate hyperkalemia owing to leukocytosis that occurs with the condition.

False increases can occur owing to situational increases in potassium in the specimen:

- Potassium is released when blood cells are destroyed (thus any crush injury or hemolysis).
- False increases are found in specimens that are left at room temperature for a few hours owing to potassium leakage from blood cells.
- False increases can result from vigorous hand pumping during the venipuncture procedure owing to hemolysis.
- Specimens collected above and IV line may be contaminated with IV fluids.
- Dehydration may cause increased levels; thus hydration status should be assessed.

The nurse should assess the heart because potassium excess can cause heart rhythm (pulse) and ECG changes, including

- Ventricular fibrillation
- Prolonged PR interval; peaked, narrow T waves; and shortened QT interval progressing to a widened/prolonged QRS complex as potassium level rises
- Cardiac muscle flaccidity with weakened contractions (owing to rapid onset of hyperkalemia or high levels of potassium)
- Cardiac arrest

Other symptoms the patient may report include such neurologic symptoms as

- Tingling in the extremities
- Weakness

- Numbness
- Paralysis

Gastrointestinal changes possibly owing to hyperactive smooth muscle also may be noted, including

- Nausea
- Intestinal colic (intermittent)
- Diarrhea

Sodium

Sodium is the major cation in the extracellular fluid and spaces. Most (95 percent) of the sodium in the body is found in the extracellular spaces and 5 percent in the intracellular space. The concentration of sodium across the cellular membrane plays an important part in neuromuscular cell activity. The nurse should be alert for conditions that might affect sodium levels and place the patient at risk for imbalance, such as

- Recent trauma, surgery, or shock that might cause fluid loss (triggers the rennin–angiotensin–aldosterone mechanism)
- Drugs that may increase sodium levels, including some of the following:
  - Anabolic steroids
  - Antibiotics
  - Clonidine
  - Corticosteroids
  - Cough medicines
  - Laxatives
  - Methyldopa
  - Estrogens
  - Carbenicillin
- Drugs that may decrease sodium levels, including:
  - Carbamazepine
  - Diuretics
  - Sodium-free IV fluids

- Sulfonylureas
- Angiotensin-converting enzyme (ACE) inhibitors
- Captopril
- Haloperidol
- Heparin
- Nonsteroidal anti-inflammatory drugs
- Tricyclic antidepressants
- Vasopressin

The nurse should review the patient's medication list and report to the physician if any of the preceding are being taken. Dietary intake also should be explored.

HYPONATREMIA

Hyponatremia, that is, a sodium level less than 134 mEq/L (134 mmol/L), most often results from excessive fluid retention or infusion that dilutes the sodium in the blood. Patients with conditions that result in excessive retention of fluid, such as the syndrome of inappropriate antidiuretic hormone (SIADH), also should be observed for a dilutional hyponatremia. Patients at highest risk for the development of hyponatremia who should be assessed closely include those experiencing neurologic procedures or with conditions that cause cerebral salt wasting (CSW) and a loss of sodium, such as subarachnoid hemorrhage and carcinoma or infection in the brain or meninges, or those taking medications that can cause sodium loss, such as antipsychotic drugs.

Nursing assessments may reveal symptoms whose severity will vary depending on the degree and speed of onset of the hyponatremia. Symptoms the nurse may observe or the patient may report include

- General fatigue
- Weakness
- Nausea
- Headache

More severe neurological symptoms may include

- Confusion
- Seizure
- Coma
- Death

HYPERNATREMIA

Hypernatremia, that is, sodium levels of 146 mEq/L (146 mmol/L) or higher, results from excessive sodium intake or sodium retention with excessive loss of water owing to diarrhea, diuretic medication use, vomiting, sweating, heavy respiration, or severe burns. Therefore, these patients are at highest risk and should be monitored closely. Elderly hospitalized patients should be watched most carefully because many have chronic diseases that may be fatal in combination with excessive sodium and fluid loss.

Symptoms the nurse may note that indicate sodium elevation, or hypernatremia, include

- Signs of dehydration
  - Dry skin and mucous membranes
  - Slow skin turgor
  - Complaints of thirst
- Neurologic changes, including
  - Twitching
  - Irritability
  - Delirium
- Symptoms similar to those found in hyponatremia, including
  - Fatigue
  - Weakness
  - Nausea
  - Headache
- In more severe cases
  - Confusion
  - Seizure
  - Coma
  - Death

Chloride

The level of chloride usually follows the sodium level, except in cases of acid–base imbalance, when chloride levels are associated with bicarbonate levels. Most of the chloride in the body comes from the salt (sodium chloride) ingested and absorbed in the intestines as food is digested. Chloride is excreted from the body in the urine. Tests for sodium, potassium, and bicarbonate usually are done at the same time as a blood test for chloride. The normal range for chloride is 97–109 mEq/L (97–109 mmol/L).

The drugs that interfere with chloride levels are those listed with sodium. A dietary history also may be beneficial.

HYPOCHLOREMIA

Low serum chloride levels, that is, less than 97 mEq/L (97 mmol/L), often result from diarrhea, vomiting, gastric suctioning (resulting in loss of acid and metabolic alkalosis), chronic respiratory disease (causing respiratory acidosis), and any condition that causes a loss of sodium owing to decreased reabsorption of sodium and chloride. Urine chloride levels may be measured to determine if the cause of hypochloremia is a loss of sodium and excess of base, such as occurs with vomiting, diuretics that show a low urine chloride level, or hormones such as cortisol or aldosterone that show a high urine chloride level.

Symptoms the nurse might note in patients with hypochloremia include

- Hyperexcitability of the muscles and nerves
- Shallow respirations
- Low blood pressure (hypotension)
- Tetany

HYPERCHLOREMIA

High serum levels of chloride (hyperchloremia), that is levels of 109 mEq/L (109 mmol/L) or higher, can result from dehydration and other conditions, including renal disease and excess parathyroid hormone (PTH). Hyperchloremia also results from metabolic acidosis owing to the loss of base and respiratory alkalosis that occurs with hyperventilation.

Symptoms the nurse might note in patients with hyperchloremia include

- Lethargy
- Weakness
- Deep breathing

Calcium

Calcium has a vital role in neuromuscular function. Total calcium levels are determined during a general admissions panel of blood work. The levels normally range from 8.9 to 10.3 mg/dL (2.23 to 2.57 mmol/L). In certain situations, ionized calcium levels, which should be between 4.65 and 5.28 mg/dL (adults), provide a better picture of whether or not adequate levels of calcium are present. This is particularly true when a protein deficiency exist because 50 percent of the calcium found in the body is bound to protein.

HYPOCALCEMIA

Low calcium levels, that is, levels of 8.4 mg/dL (2.0 mmol/L) or less, are commonly caused by low protein levels, especially low albumin, which is often present with malnutrition, particularly in alcoholics. In addition, low calcium levels can result from

- Decreased parathyroid gland function (i.e., hypoparathyroidism)
- Decreased dietary intake of calcium
- Decreased levels of vitamin D
- Magnesium deficiency
- Elevated phosphorus
- Acute inflammation of the pancreas
- Chronic renal failure
- Calcium ions becoming bound to protein (alkalosis)
- Bone disease
- Malnutrition
- Alcoholism

Low ionized calcium levels (serum calcium not bound to protein) have the same causes as low levels of chloride, except low protein, in which case the ionized calcium will be normal.

The nurse may note the following signs of hypocalcemia:

- Nervousness
- Excitability
- Tetany

HYPERCALCEMIA

Elevated serum calcium levels, that is, levels of 10.6 mg/dL (2.8 mmol/L) or higher, result most commonly from increased parathyroid function often owing to a tumor or from cancer in the bones that releases calcium into the bloodstream. Additional causes of hypercalcemia include

- Hyperthyroidism
- Bone breakage with inactivity
- Sarcoidosis
- Tuberculosis
- Vitamin D excess
- Kidney transplant

Urine calcium levels will indicate the amount of calcium being excreted in the urine. Additionally, an ionized calcium test may be performed to measure the amount of calcium that is not bound to protein in the blood. The level of ionized calcium in the blood is not affected by the amount of protein in the blood.

Symptoms the nurse might note in patients with hypercalcemia include

- Anorexia
- Nausea
- Vomiting
- Somnolence
- Coma

Magnesium

Magnesium is found primarily in the intracellular environment and is bound to adenosine triphosphate (ATP). Thus magnesium is important in almost all the body's metabolic functions. Elevated magnesium levels cause sedation and depressed neuromuscular activity, whereas low levels of magnesium cause neuromuscular excitability.

HYPOMAGNESEMIA

Decreased magnesium levels, that is, levels of 1.2 mEq/L (0.64 mmol/L) or less, may be noted in patients with conditions that cause excessive urinary loss of magnesium, including poorly controlled diabetes and alcohol abuse, or in patients using drugs such as loop and thiazide diuretics (e.g., Lasix, Bumex, Edecrin, and hydrochlorothiazide), cisplatin (which is used widely to treat cancer), and the antibiotics gentamicin, amphotericin, and cyclosporine. Hypomagnesemia also can result from conditions resulting in chronic malabsorption such as occurs with diarrhea and fat malabsorption (which usually occurs after intestinal surgery or infection) or problems such as Crohn's disease, gluten-sensitive enteropathy, and regional enteritis. Conditions that cause frequent or severe vomiting may result in a loss of magnesium as well, and toxemia in pregnancy has been associated with hypomagnesemia.

The nurse may note many symptoms, including the following signs of hypomagnesemia:

- Neuromuscular weakness
- Irritability
- Convulsions
- Tetany (owing to low calcium metabolism)
- ECG changes
- Neurologic changes, including delirium

HYPERMAGNESEMIA

Elevation of serum magnesium, that is, to levels of 2.1 mEq/L (1.06 mmol/L) or more, may result from an excessive intake of magnesium, specifically found in antacids, as well as from renal failure owing to decreased excretion of magnesium.

The nurse may note the following signs of hypermagnesemia:

- Mental status changes
- Nausea
- Diarrhea
- Appetite loss
- Muscle weakness
- Difficulty breathing
- Extremely low blood pressure
- Irregular heartbeat

Phosphate

Phosphate values are assessed to determine the amount of phosphorus in the body. Phosphate levels represent the phosphorous that is inorganic, or not part of another organic compound. Levels also may be evaluated when exploring PTH or calcium imbalances.

HYPOPHOSPHATEMIA

Low phosphate levels, that is, levels less than 3.0 mg/dL (4.0 mg/dL in children) or 0.97 mmol/L (1.45 mmol/L in children), may result from poor absorption such as occurs with ingestion of antacids that bind to phosphate. Phosphate may be decreased with reduced renal reabsorption often secondary to high levels of parathyroid hormone (PTH), which causes a retention of calcium and loss of phosphate through the kidneys, or in high calcium levels and vitamin D deficiency. Low serum phosphate levels may be noted in alkalosis because phosphate is shifted into the cells to buffer the pH.

3. The nurse may note respiratory distress in patients with hypophosphatemia owing to weakness of respiratory muscles, particularly the diaphragm, which may cause respiratory failure and difficulty in weaning the patient from mechanical ventilation, and in patients with an increased tendency for hemoglobin to cling onto oxygen, resulting in less oxygen availability to tissues. Cardiac muscle weakness with low blood pressure and dysrhythmias also may be noted, as well as neurologic symptoms, including delirium, seizures, and peripheral neuropathy.

HYPERPHOSPHATEMIA

Patients with bone cancer are at risk for hyperphosphatemia, that is, levels greater than 4.6 mg/dL (6.6 mg/dL in children) or 1.46 mmol/L (2.2 mmol/L in children), owing to the release of phosphate from the bones by tumors. Sarcoidosis; acromegaly owing to growth hormone deficiency; renal failure; cell injury such as occurs in trauma, severe infection, rhabdomyolysis, and hemolytic anemia; and conditions of hypoparathyroidism and hypocalcemia, vitamin D intoxication, hyperalimentation, thyrotoxicosis, and acidosis may predispose a patient to hyperphosphatemia.

Patients with hyperphosphatemia manifest symptoms related to the hypocalcemia and decreased vitamin D that accompanies it, in addition to signs of low phosphate.

3. The nurse may observe central nervous system (CNS) symptoms, including altered mental status with paresthesias, delirium, convulsions, seizures, and coma, as well as muscle cramping, tetany, and hyperexcitability (Chvostek and Trousseau signs). In addition, hypotension and heart failure, as well as a pronlonged QT interval, may be noted. Long-term hyperphosphatemia can result in vascular wall calcification and arteriosclerosis with increased blood pressure and ventricular hypertrophy.

Blood Urea Nitrogen and Creatinine

The level of blood urea nitrogen (BUN), a by-product of protein metabolism, is used to assess renal function and has an adult normal range of 10–20 mg/dL (3.6–7.1 mmol/L). The range for an infant or child is 5–18 mg/dL for and slightly lower for the newborn.

Creatinine is also a by-product of metabolism, and its level closely indicates renal function because the level is not affected greatly by intake but rather by renal output. Creatinine has an adult normal range of 0.5–1.1 mg/dL (44–97 mol/L). Since renal failure has a major impact on all electrolytes, it is important to view these indicators of renal function.

Conclusion

A number of laboratory tests and assessments may be performed to determine the presence of fluid and electrolyte and acid–base imbalances. The nurse should look at all data, including laboratory values and physical assessment, and evaluate them in the context of the patient's history and chronic diseases, if present. Several key points should be noted from this diagnostics chapter:

- Laboratory test results are reported using various units of measure, so the nurse must take care to evaluate such results using the correct measurement units.
- The level of fluid in the body can result in altered laboratory values and affect electrolyte levels in the body.
- Acid–base imbalances can result in electrolyte imbalances.
- Inadequate respiratory function can result in altered acid–base balance and multiple electrolyte imbalances owing to hypoxemia.
- Electrolytes affect electrically charged cells, specifically nerves and muscles, with the potential for a critical impact on heart and brain function.
- Acidosis or alkalosis can be respiratory or metabolic in origin.
- Laboratory values may indicate an acid–base imbalance originating in one system (e.g., respiratory or metabolic) with abnormal values being seen in another system as it attempts to buffer and restore the acid–base imbalance
- The nurse should monitor patients who are at risk for developing acid–base imbalance to promote early detection and treatment.

Case Situation

Alea Suarez, age 24, was admitted 2 days ago after a car accident in which she suffered a head injury with a subdural hematoma (bleeding inside the skull) and a fracture at the base of the skull. Ms. Suarez is drowsy but oriented to person, place, and time. Vital signs reveal blood pressure (BP) 100/30 mm Hg, pulse (P) 110 beats/minute (faint), respiration (R) 10 breaths/minute (shallow), and temperature (T) 36.8°C. Ms. Suarez is receiving 2 L of oxygen via nasal cannula. The nurse notes that her urine output has increased and today is averaging 250 mL/h. Diagnostic blood tests are done and reveal

Na^+ = 149 mEq/L or mmol/L

K^+ = 3.0 mEq/L or mmol/L

Cl^- = 119 mEq/L or mmol/L

CO_2 = 32 mEq/L or mmol/L

Arterial blood-gas analysis reveals

pH = 7.30

P_{CO_2} = 50 mm Hg

P_{O_2} = 80 mm Hg

HCO_3 = 31 mEq/L

Base excess = +3 mEq/L

Urinalysis showed a specific gravity of 1.010

The nurse explores the pathophysiology of head injury to determine what fluid, electrolyte, and acid–base imbalances Ms. Suarez is at risk for and discovers

- Head trauma can result in pituitary damage and can decrease or eliminate ADH release (i.e., diabetes insipidus) or can cause an increase in ADH release (i.e., SIADH).

- Respiratory controls are located in the brain and can be damaged from head trauma or from pressure buildup in the skull owing to hematoma formation.

- Disorders in sodium, potassium, and glucose may be noted owing to damage to the hypothalamus and pituitary that will affect the release of hormones that control metabolism (e.g., thyrotropin-releasing hormone [TRH] and thyroid-stimulating hormone [TSH]) and fluids and electrolytes (e.g., corticotrophin-releasing hormone [CRH] and adrenocorticotropin hormone [ACTH]).

- Aldosterone secretion may be affected, resulting in sodium, potassium, and fluid changes.
- Blood glucose levels may be affected, with possible hypoglycemia or hyperglycemia with osmotic diuresis and possible ketoacidosis.

With these thoughts in mind, the nurse would examine the test results and note

- The sodium level is high possibly owing to the diuresis and a possible lack of ADH with the head trauma. Fluid was lost but not sodium, so hemoconcentration of sodium leads to higher levels.
- Chloride level is high owing to the link with sodium concentration.
- The potassium level is low possibly owing to loss with the diuresis.
- Specific gravity shows that the osmolality of the urine is low owing to the large volumes of unconcentrated urine being produced.
- CO_2 level is high possibly owing to bicarbonate retention to balance the respiratory acid (Pco_2).
- pH shows an acidotic state.
- Pco_2 shows an elevation in respiratory acid indicating a respiratory acidosis.
- Oxygen level is at the low end of the normal range, presenting a risk for hypoxemia with lactic acidosis should hypoventilation continue or worsen.
- HCO_3 is slightly elevated; given the acidotic state, this might be the beginning of a compensatory buffering mechanism.
- Base excess indicates elevated bicarbonate, which further supports the buffering of respiratory acids.

The nurse is not surprised when the patient is diagnosed with diabetes insipidus (i.e., deficient levels of ADH) and anticipates treatment with ADH supplements and fluid replacement. The nurse will watch closely for fluid retention and possible overload in case the dose exceeds the patient's requirements. The nurse would monitor electrolytes and might anticipate potassium supplements for the hypokalemia.

The diagnosis of subdural hematoma explains the depressed respirations, which have resulted in carbon dioxide retention and respiratory acidosis. The metabolic system is beginning to buffer the respiratory acids with retention of bicarbonate. The nurse would watch the oxygen levels and respiratory rate closely and continue supplemental oxygen therapy to maintain adequate oxygenation and would prepare to artificially ventilate Ms. Suarez to improve CO_2 removal and total ventilatory effectiveness.

Final Check-up

1. Hosea, age 15 years, has had diarrhea for the past 5 days. He has been able to drink small sips of water, but any volume taken in stimulates more diarrhea. He is admitted to the hospital with suspected electrolyte imbalance. Which of the following is the nurse likely to observe?

    (a) Magnesium levels of 2.2 mEq/L or higher

    (b) Elastic and moist skin

    (c) Potassium levels of 2.5 mEq/L or lower

    (d) Dilute yellow urine output

2. If a patient is low on fluid volume, what signs might the nurse note?

    (a) High levels of sodium owing to hemoconcentration

    (b) Low levels of chloride owing to hemoconcentration

    (c) Low levels of calcium owing to renal reabsorption

    (d) High levels of magnesium owing to renal reabsorption

3. A high level of extracellular Na^+ will result in what sign or symptom?

    (a) Sedation

    (b) Slow reflex response

    (c) Irritability

    (d) Polyphagia

4. Which of the following statements is accurate about the patient at risk for a potassium imbalance?

    (a) The patient taking diuretics is at risk for hypokalemia.

    (b) The patient with high magnesium levels is at risk for hypokalemia.

    (c) Addison's disease places a patient at risk for hyperkalemia.

    (d) Aldosterone excess places a patient at risk for hyperkalemia.

5. If the nurse notes that a patient has a blood pH of 7.25 and a $Paco_2$ of 50 mm Hg, what additional observations are likely?

    (a) Slow respiratory rate

    (b) Shallow respirations

    (c) Low urinary bicarbonate levels

    (d) Numbness and muscle spasm (tetany)

References

Metheny NM. *Fluid and Electrolyte Balance: Nursing Considerations,* 4th ed. Philadelphia: Lippincott, 2000.

Pagana KD, Pagana TJ. *Mosby's Manual of Diagnostic and Laboratory Tests,* 3rd ed. St. Louis: Mosby Elsevier, 2006.

Saladin K. *Anatomy and Physiology: The Unity of Form and Function,* 4th ed. New York: McGraw-Hill, 2007.

Smeltzer S, Bare B, Hinkle J, Cheever K. *Brunner and Suddarth's Textbook of Medical-Surgical Nursing,* 11th ed. Philadelphia: Lippincott, Williams & Willams, 2008.

Web Sites

www.nephrologychannel.com/electrolytes/hypokalemia.shtml

www.ccmtutorials.com/misc/phosphate/page_05.htm

PART TWO

Fluid, Electrolyte, and Acid–Base Imbalances

CHAPTER 4

Fluid Volume Imbalances: Hypovolemia and Hypervolemia

Learning Objectives

At the end of this chapter, the student will be able to

1. Compare and contrast hypervolemia and hypovolemia.

2. Identify patients at high risk for fluid imbalance.

3. Distinguish symptoms of mild to extreme fluid imbalances.

4. Identify diagnostic values associated with fluid imbalnces.

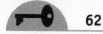
5 Discuss the potential complications related to hypervolemia and hypovolemia.

6 Determine the nursing implications related to treatments for fluid imbalances.

Key Terms

Ascites	Fluid volume deficit
Dehydration	Hydrostatic pressure
Dialysis	Oncotic pressure
Edema	Anasarca

Overview

Fluid makes up more than half the body's weight and thus plays a critical role in the function of the human body. Fluid balance is important to homeostasis. Circulation of the nutrients and oxygen in the blood is critical to maintaining life. Of the 60 percent of body weight represented by fluids for the average adult, the largest amount (40 percent) is located inside the cell (i.e., intracellular), and the remainder is extracellular fluid (20 percent), plasma (5 percent) and interstitial fluid (15 percent). Water is essential for cellular function, with many reactions in the body involving the exchange of hydrogen ions. Both an excess and a deficiency of body fluids dimish the body's ability to circulate blood effectively.

Fluid balance requires adequate intake as well as output based on fluid levels in the body. Water intake comes with liquids ingested (50 percent) and foods eaten (40 percent), as well as a small amount produced in metabolic processes (10 percent). Issues arise when patients do not take in adequate fluid or lose excessive fluids owing to

Decreased intake

- Lack of access to clean water or food
- Inability to eat or drink without assistance
- Inability to chew
- Inability to swallow
- Nausea (decreasing the desire to eat or drink)

Excess loss

- Vomiting (causing problems with hydration, nutrition, electrolytes, and acid–base balance)
- Diarrhea (causing loss of fluids and nutrients including electrolytes)
- Malabsorption (causing fluid and nutrient loss)
- Bleeding
- Fluid drainage (e.g., from wounds, nasogastric suctioning, etc.)

Problems also can arise with excessive body fluids. It is uncommon for an individual to overload his or her body with fluid in the presence of functioning kidneys that excrete excess water. However, in some neurologic conditions that migh cause an individual to drink uncontrollably, hypervolemia could occur. More commonly, excessive intake of water occurs when fluids are infused intravenously. Hypervolemia also can result when fluid output is altered, such as occurs with decreased renal function or renal failure. The normal mechanism for retaining fluid based on body need cannot function when the kidneys are unable to regulate release or retention of fluid based on body need. Regulation of body fluids was discussed in Chapter 1 and will be discussed again later in this chapter.

Normal Intake and Output

Humans normally will seek out fluids because of a thirst mechanism that induces a craving for liquids when the body needs fluid. People who cannot access the desired fluids are at risk for inadequate intake. For example, people who are stranded in areas without clean water sources are at risk for hypovolemia. Fluid deficits are also found in people who are unable to obtain food and fluids without assistance (e.g., infants, unconscious individuals, and immobile or mobility challenged individuals) and are not given adequate food and fluids.

Relatedly, an individual with a blockage (e.g., a tumor) along the oral–esophageal passage or gastrointestinal track may have difficulty ingesting and retaining adequate fluids. People with chewing difficulty may not take in inadequate fluid-containing foods. Individuals with difficulty swallowing owing to obstruction or mechanical difficulties resulting in choking and possible aspiration of fluid into the lungs may experience fluid deficits. People with a decreased desire to ingest fluids owing to nausea or a decreased thirst mechanism that occurs with aging may fail to ingest adequate fluids.

Fluid is lost normally through the kidneys or gastrointestinal tract or as a result of sweating and other insensible loss. When uncontrolled loss occurs, such as with

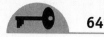
diarrhea or profuse diaphoresis (sweating), hypovolemia can result. Similarly, if fluid is lost from the body through injury resulting in blood loss or wound drainage, hypovolemia can occur.

Fluid Regulation

Fluid regulation is based on osmolality and volume triggers. As fluid is lost from the body,

- Extracellular fluid increases in osmolarity.
- Fluid is drawn from the cells to decrease plasma osmolarity.
- The increased osmolality triggers the release of antidiuretic hormone (ADH) to evoke renal retention of fluid.
- The low fluid volume triggers the renin–angiotensin–aldosterone mechanism.
- Vasoconstriction occurs around the small blood amount.
- Retention of sodium and water occurs to increase blood volume.
- The atrial natriuretic peptide (ANP) mechanism, which is usually responsible for stimulating excretion of excess fluids, is inhibited
- The thirst mechanism is stimulated to drive the individual to seek and ingest fluids to increase fluid volume in the body.

Problems arise when there is a failure or a decrease in function in any of the fluid regulation mechanisms. For example, in aging, the thirst mechanism is suppressed. The elderly patient may not drink adequate fluids owing to a lack of the thirst drive, and hypovolemia could result. Problems also arise if the regulating mechanisms fail to excrete excess water from the body, such as might occur with renal failure, and fluid overload results.

Fluid Circulation

Fluid is circulated through the body, carrying essential oxygen and nutrients to the tissues. This circulation requires effective cardiac function to pump blood into the blood vessels and maintain adequate, but not excessive, pressure inside the vessels to drive fluid out to the tissues. Adequate proteins are needed to draw fluid back into the blood vessels carrying metabolic waste for transport to the lungs, liver, and intestines and kidneys for removal from the body. The process of tissue perfusion requires a balance of pressures in the blood vessels. **Hydrostatic pressure** is the force against the blood cell imposed by the fluid volume that causes fluid to move out of the blood vessel and into the tissues. **Oncotic pressure** is the pressure exerted by the difference in concentration between the fluid inside the blood vessel and the fluid outside the blood vessel that causes fluid to move into the blood vessel from the tissues across a concentration gradient.

Hydrostatic pressure is high in arteries and low in veins, thus pushing well-oxygenated blood out of the arteries and into tissues, and the drop in pressure in the veins allows deoxygenated blood into the venous blood vessels for transport to the heart and lungs for reoxygenation. Oncotic pressure, which is lower in the arteries because blood is more dilute but higher in the more concentrated blood in the veins, is a powerful force drawing fluid back into the blood vessels (Fig. 4–1). The strongest oncotic pressure is exerted by proteins in the blood.

The pressures inside the blood cell are affected by the overall fluid volume in the body, as well as by the proteins in the body that keep fluid inside the blood vessels. Inadequate or excessive volume inside the blood vessels could hamper the circulation of fluid out to or in from the tissues. The inadequate circulation that results from fluid imbalance could cause irreversible cell damage and system failure.

Often fluid shifts will involve electrolyte changes as well. Sodium (and chloride) often will move with water; thus loss of sodium can result in loss of water, and vice versa. On occasion, drugs or hormones can cause a loss of sodium but retention of water; this causes hypervolemia and dilution of sodium content in the body, resulting in a relative hyponatremia. The fluid is hypotonic (low osmolality), causing fluid to move into cells and resulting in cellular swelling

A loss of fluid from the body without loss of sodium can lead to hypovolemia and concentration of sodium and hypernatremia. Fluid then is hypertonic and can cause cellular shrinkage owing to fluids moving out of cells in an attempt to balance the hypertonic fluid. The symptoms of fluid imbalance can be accompanied by symptoms of electrolyte imbalance and shifts in other electrolytes that occur in an attempt to balance electrolytes.

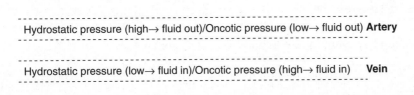

Hydrostatic pressure (high→ fluid out)/Oncotic pressure (low→ fluid out) **Artery**

Hydrostatic pressure (low→ fluid in)/Oncotic pressure (high→ fluid in)   **Vein**

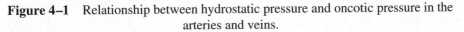

Figure 4–1   Relationship between hydrostatic pressure and oncotic pressure in the arteries and veins.

Hypovolemia

Hypovolemia is a deficiency of body fluid that results when there is a total decrease in the fluid volume in the body or a relative decrease in body fluid owing to fluid loss from the blood vessels into the tissues. Hypovolemia can be classified as **fluid volume deficit**—the loss of water and sodium from the body—or as **dehydration**—the loss of water from the body in excess of sodium, resulting in an increased osmolality. While hypovolemia has significance relative to circulatory needs, loss of fluid accompanied by changes in osmolality and sodium concentration in the body has a more profound impact on the body and survival. The detrimental result is that

- Less blood volume is available to carry critical oxygen and nutrients to the tissues.

- Loss of water could interfere with cell function.

- Electrolyte imbalance and osmolality change could accompany water loss.

- Cell shrinkage or swelling could occur depending on the osmolality change.

- If tissues such as the brain and the heart are deprived of vital circulation, tissue death can occur.

- Tissue death can be followed by organ failure and death.

Fluid volume deficit occurs in situations such as

- Hemorrhage
- Diarrhea
- Prolonged vomiting
- Severe burns
- Less commonly, aldosterone deficit (Addison's disease), in which the body loses or fails to conserve fluid and sodium, and circulating volume is decreased—the serum osmolality is essentially unchanged **5**

The low blood pressure that results from the loss of hydrostatic pressure in the blood vessels triggers the regulatory mechanisms that attempts to restore hydrostatic pressure with vasoconstriction and reserve fluid by decreasing loss through the kidneys and increasing intake. Hypovolemia stimulates

- The release of renin and then angiotensin II and eventually aldosterone

- Vasoconstriction to attempt to maintain blood pressure and circulation (renin)

- The reabsorption of sodium and water (aldosterone) to restore volume
- The thirst center in an attempt to restore volume through increased intake

In dehydration, fluid volume is also decreased, but there is an increase in the osmolality of the blood because an equivalent amount of sodium was not lost. This form of hypovolemia occurs when fluid is lost but not replaced because the individual is unable to drink (e.g., an infant, an unconscious child or adult, or someone stranded without access to drinkable water) or did not experience the normal thirst impulse (e.g., elderly persons). The result would be a loss of water without replacement and without an equal loss of sodium, resulting in an elevation in sodium concentration in the blood and increased serum osmolality. Dehydration can occur through such mechanisms as profuse sweating, diuresis (e.g., in diabetes insipidus [deficient ADH] or diabetes mellitus and osmotic fluid loss), or excessive diuretic use. **2**

CAUSES AND SYMPTOMS

The causes of hypovolemia are inadequate intake or excessive output of fluid and may include

- Fluid loss through diarrhea
- Fluid loss through vomiting
- Overuse of diuretics
- Trauma or disease of the kidney
- Blood loss
- Burns
- Edema = fluid in body tissues (e.g., anasarca or ascites)

Depending on the type of fluid loss and replacement of fluids, hypovolemia can be one of three forms (relative to the sodium loss):

- *Isotonic hypovolemia*—when water and sodium are lost, such as with diarrhea
- *Hyponatremic hypovolemia*—when water and sodium are lost, but only water is partially replaced without an equivalent sodium replacement
- *Hypernatremic hypovolemia*—when water and sodium are, lost but only sodium is replaced with insufficient water replacement

The body has compensatory mechanisms to maintain circulation to vital organs for as long as possible and sends messages to stimulate the individual to take in fluids, such as thirst, and to reserve fluids through the kidneys and bowel. If fluid is not restored in a timely manner, severe damage can occur to tissues as compensatory mechanisms begin to fail.

3 Symptoms and compensatory mechanisms for hypovolemia include the following:

- Vasoconstriction maintains the blood pressure (hydrostatic pressure) needed to propel fluid containing needed oxygen and nutrients out of the blood vessels and into the tissues.

- Vasoconstriction shifts blood from certain areas of the body, such as the skin and gastrointestinal tract, which are considered less critical areas, to provide circulation to the brain and other vital tissues.

- An additional automatic response decreases perfusion to the kidneys. This serves multiple purposes, including decreasing loss of fluids through the urine; thus urinary output decreases, signaling a low fluid volume.

- As compensatory mechanism begin to fail, neurologic symptoms such as confusion, irritability, and progressive loss of consciousness may manifest.

- The low perfusion pressure to the kidneys triggers feedback mechanisms such as the renin–angiotensin–aldosterone system to stimulate vasoconstriction and reabsorption of sodium and water in an attempt to increase fluid volume.

Although urine output will vary among individuals, the minimum output of 30 mL/h (less in infants and children) is used to gauge adequate renal perfusion and function, but high urine outputs can occur in the presence of certain types of renal failure, so this is not always a conclusive measure.

The limited fluid volume results in decreased stroke volume in the heart. In order to maintain cardiac output, the heart rate increases:

$$CO \text{ (cardiac output)} = SV \text{ (stroke volume)} \times HR \text{ (heart rate)}$$

Thus tachycardia occurs. In addition, to maximize the oxygenation of the little blood that is circulating, and because the tissues will become hypoxic, resulting in a metabolic acidosis, the respiratory system will be triggered to increase respiratory rate, and thus tachypnea is noted.

Compensatory mechanisms can last for a time but are costly owing to the increased workload placed on the heart and lungs at a time when limited nutrients are being delivered to tissues. The speed of onset of hypovolemia is important because patients with rapid fluid loss will have limited opportunity for compensatory mechanisms to slow the impact of the fluid deficit. The underlying problem must be corrected to reverse the hypovolemia before compensatory mechanisms fail.

Types and Causes of Hypovolemia

A common cause of true hypovolemia is dehydration owing to inadequate intake of fluids, excessive loss of fluids, or a combination of the two. Dehydration is a true danger in the elderly because the thirst mechanism, which stimulates one to drink fluids, is diminished with age. Additionally, children, whose total-body fluid content is high and have high fluid needs, can dehydrate more quickly than adults if they are ill and nausea or gastrointestinal upset causes them to refuse fluid intake. **2**

Additional causes of hypovolemia include loss of fluids through

- Perspiration
- Vomiting
- Diarrhea

These conditions occur often in conjunction with infection or another condition that causes patients to refuse oral intake and will compound the dehydration experienced.

Blood loss through slow, prolonged bleeding or rapid bleeding also will cause hypovolemia. The degree and duration of the decreased fluid intake, prolonged vomiting or diarrhea, or blood loss will determine the severity of the hypovolemia and the amount of fluids needed to restore volume.

Relative hypovolemia can occur when a large portion of the body's fluids escape into the tissues, most often owing to low oncotic pressures as a result of decreased protein. The circulating blood volume is decreased, which reduces venous return and results in symptoms similar to those of inadequate intake or fluid loss from the body. Symptoms of hypovolemia can occur when the total volume of fluid in the body is adequate. If an excess amount of fluid volume remains in the tissues, decreased volume in the blood vessels will result.

Relatedly, if the fluid in the blood vessels pools owing to vasodilation, which decreases hydrostatic pressure in the arteries, blood volume circulating through the vessels and moving out to the tissues is decreased, and symptoms of hypovolemia result (Fig. 4–2).

Arteries Hydrostatic pressure (low due to pooled volume)/**Veins** (higher than normal) blood pools…blood pools- → slow blood flow/slow venous reabsorption → *Edema in tissues*

Figure 4–2 Relationship between hydrostatic pressure and blood flow in the arteries and veins.

Thus any condition that reduces the protein level in the blood will cause fluids to remain in the tissues. This causes massive edema and a reduction in circulating blood volume. In addition, any condition that causes massive vasodilation, for example, a systemic infection (sepsis), can cause a relative hypovolemia. In sepsis,

- Massive vasodilatation occurs
- Blood pools
- Blood fails to circulate

The compensatory mechanisms described earlier will be seen. However, as stated earlier, these mechanisms can sustain life for only a limited time, and the hypovolemic state and underlying cause must be resolved.

Symptoms of Hypovolemia

The compensatory mechanisms include decreasing perfusion to the kidneys to preserve volume and other mechanisms that result in such symptoms as

- Oliguria
- Skin feeling cool to touch owing to constriction of skin blood vessels
- Tachycardia in an attempt to circulate more blood
- Tachypnea in an attempt to increase the oxygen supply to the tissues
- Decreased capillary refill (> 5 seconds)
- Dry mucous membranes (e.g., a dry tongue)
- Orthostatic hypotension (i.e., dizziness on standing up from a seated or reclining position owing to a drop in cerebral blood pressure)
- Cool extremities (e.g., cool fingers)
- Blanching of skin, which will result in a prolonged pallor
- Dry skin
- A weak pulse
- Decreased skin turgor (i.e., when the skin is pinched, it will reveal a slow return to original position)

Table 4–1 provides a summary of the symptoms of hypovolemia.

As stated in chapter 3, laboratory values often will reveal an elevated hematocrit, high specific gravity, and increased osmolarity. Initially, the blood pressure may remain within normal range or even may be slightly elevated owing to compensatory vasoconstriction, but as compensatory mechanisms fail, blood pressure will decrease. If blood pressure drops below a certain level, the hydrostatic pressure

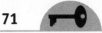

Table 4–1   Symptoms of Hypovolemia

Confusion, decreased sensorium
Stomach: Decreased bowel sounds
Skin (arms, trunk, and legs): Coos and pale
Kidney: Decreased urine output, concentrated urine

within the blood vessels (i.e., perfusion pressure) will be too low to send fluid out of the blood vessels to perfuse the tissues. 1

NURSING IMPLICATIONS IN TREATMENT

Treatment of the underlying problem is critical to resolution of hypovolemia.

- If blood loss has occurred, one or more blood transfusions may be given.
- If dehydration has occurred, fluid volume may be restored orally or through intravenous fluids.
- Often fluid loss in accompanied by electrolyte loss (e.g., with perspiration, vomiting, or diarrhea); thus fluid replacement includes electrolyte replacement as well.
- If the hypovolemia is relative and related to fluid moving into the tissues owing to a lack of protein and osmotic pressure in vessels, treatment will center on increasing protein (i.e., infusing albumin) in the blood vessels to bring volume into the blood vessels from the tissues.
- If blood volume is pooled, treatment may focus on eliminating the sepsis that causes the vasodilation so that blood pressure is restored.
- While treating sepsis, fluids may be given.

The nurse must monitor the patient closely during and after fluid replacement therapy because as fluid returns to the blood vessels from the tissues or as blood vessels constrict to normal diameter, fluid volume overload can result.

SPEED BUMP

1. *Which of the following patients would be at greatest risk for organ damage owing to hypovolemia?*

    (a) An 80-year-old man with slow blood loss of 1 pint over 5 months

    (b) A 5-year-old child with diarrhea for the past 3 hours

    (c) A 50-year-old woman with urinary output of 300 mL/h for 4 days

    (d) A 20-year-old woman with nausea and vomiting over the last 24 hours

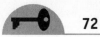
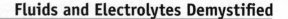

2. *Which of the following symptoms indicate a complication that is likely to occur with prolonged hypovolemia?*

 (a) *Cardiac failure owing to workload from high cardiac output*

 (b) *Respiratory depression owing to decreased stimulation of the breathing impulse*

 (c) *Edema in the extremities and abdomen owing to fluid movement into the tissues*

 (d) *Increased blood levels of waste products owing to decreased renal perfusion*

3. *The nurse suspects that Mrs. Grendal is hypovolemic. What data would support this suspicion?*

 (a) *A decreased respiratory rate*

 (b) *An elevated pulse rate*

 (c) *A decreased osmolarity*

 (d) *An elevated urinary output*

4. *What treatment would be most appropriate for a patient with hypovolemia owing to massive sepsis?*

 (a) *Blood and blood product transfusion*

 (b) *Vasopressors such as epinephrine*

 (c) *Vasodilators such as nitroglycerin*

 (d) *Diuretics such as furosemide*

Hypervolemia

Hypervolemia is an overload of body fluid that results when there is an excessive intake or decreased excretion of fluids. When the total volume of fluid in the body is increased, the workload on the heart and the pressure on the blood vessels are increased. As the hydrostatic pressure in the arterial blood vessels is increased,

- The pressure in the veins remains higher than normal.
- The fluid that was driven out into the tissues from the arteries is drawn back into the veins to a lesser degree.
- The increased fluid in the tissues results in edema.
- If the volume circulating becomes too excessive, the heart may become unable to handle the extra workload, and congestive heart failure could result.

Patients with weakened hearts, including the elderly, who often have decreased cardiac capacity to adapt to volume changes, or pediatric patients, who have smaller hearts with less capacity to handle large volumes, are at particular risk for cardiac overload. **2** Increased fluid volume also could cause a dilutional hyponatremia. Thus symptoms of low sodium concentration with fluid shifts including cerebral edema could occur. **4**

TYPES AND CAUSES OF HYPERVOLEMIA

Conditions that result in hypervolemia that involve excessive oral fluid intake are not common. A more likely cause of excessive fluid intake is accidental excessive infusion of fluids during intravenous therapy or during surgery resulting in overload. The most common conditions resulting in hypervolemia, however, include

- Insufficient renal function
- Failure of the renal system

When kidney tissue is damaged, the selective function governing excretion of fluid into the urine to control blood volume fails to function, and excessive fluid is retained with overload resulting.

Less common conditions include

- Tumors
- Central nervous system (CNS) disorders
- Pulmonary disorders
- Drugs

These conditions may result in excess fluid retention through an endocrine condition called the *syndrome of inappropriate antidiuretic hormone secretion* (SIADH). These less common conditions result in retention of water and secretion of sodium, leading to a hypervolemia with hyponatremia. **1** **2**

SYMPTOMS OF HYPERVOLEMIA

Signs and symptoms indicating the presence of hypervolemia include

- Signs of cardiac failure/congestive heart failure owing to fluid overload
  - Rales in the lungs
  - Jugular vein distension
  - Systemic edema (i.e., anasarca = total body tissue edema or swelling)

- Fluid buildup in the abdominal cavity (i.e., **ascites** = fluid in abdominal cavity)
- Weight gain owing to the high fluid volume
- Decreased perfusion to the kidneys owing to heart failure
- Decreased renal output
- Urinary output, if kidneys are functional (without SIADH), may be slightly increased, particularly as cardiac failure resolves and perfusion to kidneys is fully restored
- Symptoms of hyponatremia, such as anorexia, nausea, and malaise
- Neurologic symptoms ranging from headache to coma owing to electrolyte imbalance and fluid shifts with cerebral edema

NURSING IMPLICATIONS IN TREATMENT

6 The treatment of hypervolemia involves diuretics if kidney function is sufficient. The nurse must

- Monitor intake and output continuously.
- Monitor weight daily.
- Watch for signs of electrolyte imbalances that may result from diuretic therapy: **4**
  - Hypokalemia
  - Hyponatremia
  - Hypophophatemia
  - Hypercalcemia
  - Hypomagnesemia
- Assess signs of dehydration and hypovolemia, including
  - Poor skin turgor
  - Dry mucous membranes
  - Orthostatic hypotention
  - Decreased urine volume (< 30 mL/h)
  - Dark yellow, concentrated urine

For some patients, dialysis is needed to remove the excess fluid. **Dialysis**, the filtering of blood through an artificial kidney (or the peritoneal lining) to remove excess fluid and waste products, can be performed directly through hemodialysis with rapid filtration or through peritoneal dialysis with slower filtration across the peritoneal lining. Fluid shifts will affect blood pressure and tissue perfusion; thus the speed of dialysis is important and will have an impact on the symptoms of distress noted because of the rapid fluid and electrolyte shifts. The nurse must monitor for signs of fluid overload prior to the procedure and for signs of fluid deficit, as well as electrolyte deficit, after the procedure.

The primary electrolyte imbalance associated with the hypovolemia, a loss of sodium (i.e., hyponatremia), may require sodium infusions until the underlying condition has been resolved. Since electrolytes may shift in response to sodium imbalances, other replacements may be indicated (see Chapter 5).

The nurse should monitor for patient response to treatment, particularly noting laboratory values and vital signs. It is most important to monitor intake and output and to note signs of hypovolemia that might occur if the degree of volume overload is overestimated and the treatment is excessive. Hold diuretics until the primary-care provider is consulted. **6**

Conclusion

Fluid volume imbalance has great implications for a patient. Excess or insufficient fluid volume could result in poor tissue perfusion. Some patients are at high risk for imbalance owing to young or extreme age or preexisting conditions, such as infection or gastrointestinal upset. The causes of hypovolemia or hypervolemia vary from altered intake—insuffient or excessive intake—to altered fluid reabsorption or excretion. Key points in this chapter include

- Body fluid is critical to life.
- Circulation of body fluid depends on cardiac function and maintaining adequate pressure in blood vessels.
- Hydrostatic pressure results from fluid volume and pushes fluid out into tissues.
- Oncotic pressure relates to the concentration of intravascular fluids that pulls fluid back into the veins.
- Hypovolemia can result from excessive diuresis or insufficient fluid intake.
- Hypervolemia can result from insufficient fluid excretion owing to renal failure or hormonal imbalance.
- Hypovolemia can be relative if fluid escapes into the tissues or pools in dilated blood vessels.
- Treatment of one fluid imbalance could result in the opposite imbalance if care is not exercised.

Final Check-up

1. Pete, a 5-year-old patient, is admitted to the emergency room with a history of vomiting and diarrhea over the past 3 days. His mother is concerned because she noticed that Pete is less awake and less active than usual and will not even watch his favorite television program. Vital signs reveal a blood pressure of 70/20 mm Hg, a pulse rate of 140 beats/minute, and a respiratory rate of 45 breaths/minute. The nurse is concerned that a fluid imbalance is present. Which of the following findings would the nurse likely observe that would support the concerns regarding fluid imbalance?

   (a) Urine output is 40 mL/h.

   (b) The patient is awake and alert.

   (c) The skin is loose and nonelastic.

   (d) The skin is cool to the touch.

2. Which of the following questions would provide the most important data to further support the nurse's concerns?

   (a) What has Pete eaten today?

   (b) Which television program does Pete like the most?

   (c) What type of activities does Pete usually participate in?

   (d) What has Pete had to drink over the last 3 days?

3. The nurse would anticipate what treatment initially for Pete?

   (a) A high-protein diet

   (b) Push 50–100 mL of fluids hourly

   (c) Sodium infusions over 3 days

   (d) Antibiotics in intravenous fluids

4. Which would be the most accurate explanation for Pete's vital sign readings?

   (a) Pete is lethargic owing to the dilutional hyponatremia.

   (b) The elevated blood pressure is due to increased hydrostatic pressure.

   (c) Pete's decreased pulse rate is due to decreased circulating blood.

   (d) The respiratory rate is increased to compensate for poor circulation.

5. The nurse would monitor for what signs to prevent the treatment provided to Pete from being excessive?

(a) Pete begins to watch the television in his room.

(b) The nurse hears rales in Pete's lung fields.

(c) Pete's urine output remains at 50 mL/h for 3 hours.

(d) Skin turgor testing reveals a slow return to normal position.

References

Saladin K. *Anatomy and Physiology: The Unity of Form and Function,* 4th ed. New York: McGraw-Hill, 2007.

Pagana KD, Pagana TJ. *Mosby's Manual of Diagnostic and Laboratory Tests,* 3rd ed. St. Louis: Mosby Elsevier, 2006.

Needham A. *Comparative and Environmental Physiology Acidosis and Alkalosis.* 2004.

Web Site

http://en.wikipedia.org/wiki/Acidosis

CHAPTER 5

Sodium Imbalances: Hyponatremia and Hypernatremia

Learning Objectives

At the end of this chapter, the student will be able to

1. Compare and contrast hyponatremia and hypernatremia.
2. Identify patients at high risk for sodium imbalance.
3. Distinguish symptoms of excess and deficient sodium levels.
4. Identify diagnostic values associated with sodium imbalances.

5 Discuss the potential complications related to hyponatremia and hypernatremia.

6 Determine the nursing implications related to treatments for sodium imbalances.

Key Terms

Aldosterone

Diuresis

Edema

Hyponatremia

Hypernatremia

Osmolality

Polyruria

Overview

Sodium is the most abundant cation in the extracellular fluid and is the major factor in extracellular **osmolality** (the concentration of particles dissolved in blood). Sodium commonly moves with water, and water moves with sodium; thus, as a determinant of osmolality, the concentration of sodium has an impact on the flow of water across the cell membrane. Additionally, the concentration of sodium and volume of water play a critical role in blood pressure.

Sodium also plays an important role in nerve impulse generation and transmission. As a part of the sodium–potassium pump, the difference between the potassium and sodium concentrations is maintained through active transport across the cell membrane as needed with the help of adenosine triphosphate (ATP) as an energy source. The flow of sodium and potassium across the cell membrane of electrically charged cells results in depolarization. Thus sodium is important for nerve and muscle function. As such, sodium imbalances can affect cardiac and respiratory muscle function as well as mobility.

Sodium also plays a role in acid–base balance. Sodium binds well to chloride and bicarbonate and thus plays a part in the metabolic buffer system, preventing a strong acid from greatly affecting the pH of the blood by changing it to a weak acid.

$$\underset{\text{strong acid}}{HCl} + \underset{\text{strong base}}{NaH_2CO_3} \rightarrow \underset{\text{salt}}{NaCl} + \underset{\text{weak acid}}{H_2CO_3}$$

Thus sodium plays an important role in fluid balance, neuromuscular function, and acid–base balance. Excessive or inadequate concentrations of sodium can severely disrupt body function.

Sodium is absorbed in the intestines from foods and fluids ingested, as well as from many medications. The intake of sodium commonly far exceeds the needs of the human body, but an individual with healthy kidneys seldom will experience a buildup because excess sodium is excreted by the kidneys as needed to restore balance. A few basic facts about sodium concentration in the body include the following:

- The normal range of sodium is 135–145 mEq/L or 135 mmol/L (SI units). This reflects the concentration of sodium—the amount of sodium in relation to water (not specifically the total amount of sodium in the body).

- Sodium occurs in many different forms—sodium chloride (NaCl), sodium bicarbonate ($NaHCO_3$), and sodium phosphate (Na_2HPO_4). However, for the body to use these forms of sodium, they must be completely dissolved in water or the juices of the foods that we eat.

- The bones contain about 40 percent of the sodium found in the body; the cells of various organs contain about 2 to 5 percent, and the blood plasma and other extracellular fluids contain 55 percent.

- It has been estimated that the blood plasma normally contains about 140 mEq/L of sodium, which is higher than that found in other extracellular fluids, causing sodium to contribute greatly to the osmolality of body fluids.

The unequal distribution of sodium in the intracellular and extracellular fluids maintains an electrochemical gradient that is vital to normal functions of the body and is maintained through active transport using the sodium–potassium pump. Since sodium ions are necessary to maintain fluid levels, normal blood pressure, proper nerve impulse conduction, and the passage of nutrients into the cell, maintaining proper sodium balance is critical to life.

Sodium Regulation

The kidneys and the intestines play an important role in adjusting dietary sodium when it is too high or too low on a daily basis. Under normal conditions in the intestines.

- Sodium is absorbed from the foods that we eat, and the kidneys excrete about an equivalent amount into the urine, and as a result, sodium balance is maintained.

- If for some reason sodium intake is low, then the intestines will increase absorption, and the kidneys will reduce sodium release into the urine.

- Gastrointestinal contents contain a significant amount of sodium, and loss through suctioning, diarrhea, or vomiting could cause hyponatremia.

- Deficient intake of sodium is rare as the solitary cause of hyponatremia, and sodium loss through sweating is usually minimal. However, either of the two in combination with other risk factors can result in hyponatremia.

The regulation of sodium through the kidneys is influenced by a number of factors. The two major functions that are involved in the concentration of sodium in the blood are

- The amount of sodium itself

- The amount of water in the circulatory system

As sodium is absorbed, water will follow passively. Even though the body uses separate mechanisms to regulate these two factors (water and sodium), they work together to regulate blood pressure to normal levels. If the concentration of sodium is too low (i.e., **hyponatremia**), it can be corrected by either decreasing the water in the body or increasing sodium. When the concentration of sodium is too high (i.e., **hypernatremia**), it is corrected by absorbing less and excreting more sodium and by retaining water.

Hormones also play a vital role in maintaining the sodium level within proper balance. The triple As of sodium are

- *Antidiuretic hormone* (ADH)—which controls the reabsorption of water, which might cause a concentration or dilution of sodium.

- **Aldosterone**—which stimulates the kidneys to reabsorb sodium and reduce loss of sodium.

- *Atrial natriuretic peptide* (ANP)—which is secreted when the heart walls are stretched owing to rising blood pressure and causes sodium excretion by decreasing renal absorption, thus increasing the loss of sodium through the kidneys.

High fluid volume and increased blood pressure cause a stretch of the cardiac atrium, stimulating the release of ANP, which stimulates the kidney to excrete sodium (water follows) and leads to increased **diuresis** (high urinary output) of water and sodium, resulting in a reduced blood volume.

Table 5–1 presents a summary of the body's response to sodium excess and fluid overload.

The hormonal controls of fluid volume and sodium concentration are important to the maintenance of fluid and electrolyte balance. Disruption in the body's ability to regulate sodium and fluid can result in hypernatremia or hyponatremia.

Table 5–1   Body Response to Sodium Excess and Fluid Overload: Hormonal Responses

Gland Affected	Aldosterone: Adrenal Gland Response	ADH: Pituitary Gland Response	ANP: Heart
Sodium concentration Fluid volume Potassium concentration	Low sodium concentration, low fluid volume, or high potassium concentration → adrenal cortex secretes aldosterone → renal tubules increase sodium reabsorption and increase potassium secretion → decreased Na^+ and water excreted in urine and increased K^+ in the urine	High Na^+ concentration and high plasma osmolality stimulates posterior lobe of pituitary gland to secrete ADH → kidneys to reabsorb more water (independent of sodium) → decreased plasma osmolality → decreased sodium concentration kidneys → ADH also stimulates thirst resulting in increased oral intake of fluids → decreased serum osmolality	Right atrial distension owing to increased volume stimulates release of ANP → stimulates kidneys to increase sodium excretion and inhibits ADH and renin production → blocks action of angiotensin II on adrenal gland → no aldosterone secretion, causes relaxation of the afferent arterioles, increasing the glomerular filtration rate → high urine output → decreased fluid volume
Sodium concentration Fluid volume Potassium concentration	Low potassium concentration or high volume and ANP release → inhibits aldosterone release → kidneys excrete more water and sodium → retain, potassium	Low sodium concentration → inhibits ADH release → kidney excrete more water → raises sodium concentration	Low fluid volume results in no distension of the right atrium, thus no release of ANP

Nursing assessments that support the detection and care planning for patients with suspected sodium imbalance involve taking a history related to sodium intake, including

- An interview of the patient for a detailed medication history
  - Include prescription and over-the-counter (OTC) drugs because some may precipitate hyponatremia (e.g., antipsychotics).
- A dietary history with reference to salt, protein, and water intake is useful.
- Review patient records to determine what parenteral fluids were administered for patients who are hospitalized.

- Assess the patient's acute conditions (i.e., trauma, infections, etc.) or chronic conditions (e.g., comorbidities), particularly cardiac, pulmonary, and neurologic conditions. This assessment will assist in determining new and significant symptoms and possible sources of the imbalance.

- Intake and output are critical to detection of sodium and fluid imbalances and to implement interventions.

- All intake and output are important to determine sodium loss and gains; thus gastrointestinal and wound losses should be noted, as well as intake of candies, snacks, and other foods.

- Weights are also important as measures of fluid imbalance.

- Laboratory testing (such as osmolality) is important to help distinguish between hypervolemic or hypovolemic hyponatremia or hypernatremia.

- Urine sodium may be determined, as well as serum sodium to quantify sodium loss.

Having as complete a picture as possible can assist in proper diagnosis of the patient situation and in planning for effective interventions. **6**

Hypernatremia

Hypernatremia is elevation of the serum sodium concentration higher than 145 mEq/L. **4** Because sodium is an electrolyte that helps with nerve and muscle function, and also helps to maintain blood pressure, excessive concentrations of sodium can severely disrupt body function. Severe hypernatremia, that is, a sodium concentration above 152 mEq/L, can result in seizure and death. **5** Hypernatremia can result from

- Excessive intake from ingestion of unintentional sodium sources or excess infusion of sodium (i.e., treatment of acidosis with excessive sodium bicarbonate or high-sodium hypertonic intravenous fluids).

- Excessive ingestion of high-sodium solutions, such as sea water, or medications containing sodium (rarely causes hypernatremia because of the intestinal control of absorption of sodium).

- Decreased intake of fluids—the elderly are at risk for hypernatremia owing to a decreased thirst mechanism that results in decreased fluid intake and dehydration.

- Loss of too much water in relation to the amount of sodium in the blood.
  - This water loss can occur with **polyuria** high urinary output (i.e., the kidneys excrete too much urine).

Various causes are detailed in the discussion below.

85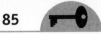

CAUSES AND SYMPTOMS

Diuretics that cause the kidneys to excrete more water than sodium are a common cause of hypernatremia. Additionally, pathology of the pituitary or hypothalamus can result in a deficiency of ADH, resulting in diabetes insipidus and excessive diuresis (with extremely high urine output).

- ADH, also called *vasopression,* is made by the hypothalamus.
- ADH then is released by the pituitary gland into the bloodstream.
- This hormone acts on the distal portion of the kidney tubule to prevent water loss from the blood into the urine.
- Inhibition of vasopression will cause the body to release more water into the urine.
- This will result in a higher plasma sodium concentration.
- Thus hypernatremia occurs in diabetes insipidus because the disease causes excessive urine production and dehydration. ❷

This disorder should not be confused with diabetes mellitus, which results from decreased or a lack of insulin production. Diabetes insipidus is casued by either failure of the hypothalamus to make vasopressin or failure of the distal portion of the kidney tubule to respond to vasopressin. The consequence of either of these two disorders is that the kidney is able to retain and regulate the body's sodium levels but is not able to retain and conserve water.

Patients who are unconscious (comatose) and are unable to drink water may suffer from hypernatremia because water is lost continually by evaporation from the lungs and urine, leading to dehydration, which causes sodium concentration to increase. Or hypernatremia can be caused by fluid loss from the body owing to excessive sweating during intense heat or exercise or loss of gastric contents, which contain significant sodium content, through prolonged diarrhea, vomiting, or simply by not drinking enough water. Any disease in which the thirst impulse is impaired is likely to cause dehydration and hypernatremia. If patients are infused with solutions containing high sodium content; such as sodium bicarbonate for treatment of acidosis, hypernatremia may occur accidentally. ❷

In hypernatremia, fluid moves out of the cells in an attempt to dilute the high concentration of sodium in the extracellular fluid. This causes cell dehydration with shrinkage, resulting in dry tissues, particularly evident in mucous membranes, loss of skin elasticity (turgor), and thirst (stimulated by ADH release).

Some symptoms of hypernatremia may vary depending on the underlying cause. If dehydration is present owing to vomiting or diarrhea or failure to drink fluids, the urine output will be low (<30 mL/h) with dark yellow appearance. However, if a hyperosmotic state or a condition causing decreased ADH release, such as diabetes insipidus, is

present, urine output may be extremely elevated. In either case, signs of dehydration will be present, including dry mucous membranes and thirst. **3** **5**

Hypernatremia can affect brain cells and cause neurologic damage, resulting in

- Confusion
- Paralysis of the muscles of the lungs
- Coma
- Even death **3** **5**

How severe the symptoms are will be directly related to how rapidly the hypernatremia developed. Hypernatremia that comes on rapidly does not allow the cells of the brain time to adapt to their new high-sodium environment and will result in with severe symptoms quickly.

NURSING IMPLICATIONS IN TREATMENT OF HYPERNATREMIA

If dehydration is the underlying cause of hypernatremia, the primary treatment will be rehydration. Of particular concern is the rate of rehydration and use of hypotonic solutions. The nurse must take care to

- Avoid overhydration, which could result in dilutional hyponatremia.
- Verify the fluids being given and avoid large volumes of hypotonic fluids.
- Infuse fluids slowly, particularly if hypernatremia has been present for an extended period. Brain tissue has adjusted to the hypernatremia and may respond to hypotonic infusions with swelling and increased intracranial pressure.
- Slow the fluid infusion and notify the primary-care provider if the patient's symptoms worsen instead of improving with rehydration.

If hormone imbalance is present, treatment centers around restoring hormone status. For example, in hyperaldosteronism, the offending tumor or tissue is removed, and in Cushing syndrome (with corticosteroids that behave like aldosterone causing absorption of sodium), treatment centers on decreasing the excess aldosterone or corticosteroids. If the level of aldosterone or corticosteroids is severely limited in the body, a deficiency of either hormone could occur, resulting in hyponatremia. **6**

In diabetes insipidus (i.e., decreased ADH secretion), supplemental ADH is provided. Care must be taken during treatment with supplement to avoid excess ADH intake, which will cause retention of water and potential for dilutional hyponatremia. **6**

SPEED BUMP

1. Which of the following clinical information indicates that the patient is at risk for hypernatremia?

    (a) Urine output over the last 8 hours was 400 mL/h.

    (b) Arterial blood-gas analysis reveals a pH above 7.50.

    (c) Water is infused intravenously at 300 mL/h.

    (d) Patient reports having nausea and vomiting for the last 4 days.

2. Which of the following pieces of information in the patient's history would alert the nurse to watch the patient closely for signs of hypernatremia?

    (a) The patient was diagnosed with chronic renal failure 6 years ago.

    (b) The patient is taking furosemide (Lasix) three times a day.

    (c) The patient's dietary history reveals a low intake of salt in foods and drinks.

    (d) The patient's occupation history indicates work outside in intense heat.

3. The nurse would monitor for which of the following signs that the treatment provided to a patient for hypernatremia may be excessive?

    (a) The patient has dry mucous membranes and complains of thirst.

    (b) The nurse hears hyperactive bowel sounds in all quadrants of the patient's abdomen.

    (c) The nurse notes that the patient's urine output is 10 mL/h for 3 hours.

    (d) The patient demonstrates weakness, confusion, and lethargy.

Hyponatremia

Decreased serum sodium concentration (i.e., **hyponatremia**) occurs when the sodium concentration in the blood plasma falls below the normal range (< 134 mEq/L). The concentration of sodium in the blood can fall because. **4**

- The total level of sodium is decreased relative to the amount of water in the body.

- The sodium level is unchanged, but the water level is increased, causing a dilution of sodium (i.e., dilutional hyponatremia).

- A combination of reduced intake of sodium or an abnormally large output of sodium also can occur.

An excessive intake of water or excessive retention of water without equivalent intake or retention of sodium can result in hyponatremia, particularly if the mechanisms that control fluid and electrolyte balance are impaired. Altered function of an organ or the hormones that regulate sodium and water (e.g., kidney, pituitary gland and hypothalamus [aldosterone] or adrenal gland [ADH] as well as ANP from the right atria) can cause excess loss of sodium or retention of water and thus can result in hyponatremia.

There are several types of hyponatremia, depending on the level of fluid in the blood:

- *Hypovolemic hypotonic hyponatremia*—fluid and solute loss, with more sodium than water lost so that the remaining body fluid is hypotonic (dilute). May occur in hemorrhage or loss of vascular volume owing to gastrointestinal or renal loss (particularly owing to diuretic use).

- *Hypervolemic hypotonic hyponatremia*—increase in water without an equal increase in sodium. Occurs with cirrhosis, hypoproteinemia (low albumin), heart failure, and nephrotic syndrome.

- *Normovolemic hypotonic hyponatremia*—occurs in hospitalized patients, particularly with increased ADH production.

In hyponatremia, fluid moves from the extracellular fluid into the cells, moving from a lower osmolality with low sodium concentrations to a higher osmolality and high sodium concentrations. This results in tissue swelling or **edema** in many body, areas and organs including the brain (Fig. 5–1).

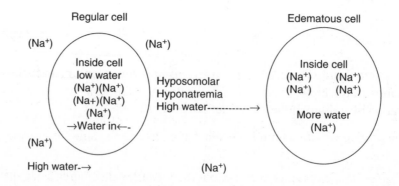

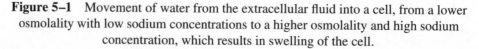

Figure 5–1   Movement of water from the extracellular fluid into a cell, from a lower osmolality with low sodium concentrations to a higher osmolality and high sodium concentration, which results in swelling of the cell.

CAUSES AND SYMPTOMS

Reduced intake of sodium, such as occurs with a low-salt diet for prolonged periods of time, can pose a threat to the body's ability to obtain adequate levels of sodium. Loss of sodium through use of some diuretics also can result in hyponatremia. These conditions by themselves may not be enough to cause low sodium, but under certain conditions, they can. For example, the patient taking diuretic drugs who also maintain a low-sodium diet would be at high risk for hyponatremia. In addition, some diarrheal diseases can cause an excessive loss of sodium. **2**

Drinking or infusing excess water is another cause of hyponatremia because excess water can dilute the sodium in the blood. For example, beer, which is mainly water and low in sodium, can lead to hyponatremia if taken in excess. Loss of sodium and water through perspiration and replacement of lost volume with water alone can result in hyponatremia. **2** The body normally will excrete the excess fluid and increase absorption of sodium to restore balance.

Relatedly, malfunction of one of the sodium–water control mechanisms, such as a kidney that normally excretes excess water, can result in fluid retention and dilutional hyponatremia. The pituitary gland and hypothalamus function to release ADH (which controls water reabsorption), and the cortex of the adrenal gland secretes aldosterone (which controls sodium reabsorption). An alteration in the function of either of these hormone systems will alter the body's regulation of sodium or water and can result in hyponatremia. **2** For example, in the syndrome of inappropriate antidiuretic hormone (SIADH), excessive ADH is produced (usually by a tumor or some pulmonary diseases such as tuberculosis or bacterial pneumonia), and the kidneys reabsorb excessive fluids, resulting in dilutional hyponatremia. Conditions causing decreased aldosterone secretion include

- Addison's disease because the adrenal cortex is not functional
- Toxemia of pregnancy
- Myxedema (i.e., hypothyroidism with hyposecretion of glucocorticoids/cortisone, which function like aldosterone)
- Estrogen-secreting tumor (similarly causes water retention and edema) **2**

Many symptoms of hyponatremia are associated with the hypotonic hydration—the presence of high water content without equivalent sodium. The most common symptoms include

- Headache
- Nausea
- Disorientation
- Tiredness
- Muscle cramps

The neurologic symptoms are believed to be caused by movement of water into brain cells, thus causing them to swell and disrupt normal functioning. The muscle cramps may occur as a result of disruption of the sodium and potassium electrolytes or of water shifting into the cell. **3**

NURSING IMPLICATIONS IN TREATMENT OF HYPONATREMIA

The primary treatment for hyponatremia owing to excess free water in the body is to remove the excess water and, if indicated, to treat the source of water retention. If diuretics are used to remove water, the nurse must monitor intake and output and electrolytes closely. Most diuretics work by removing sodium and water; thus sodium levels may remain low initially. If the patient is symptomatic, sodium supplement may be given. The nurse should monitor for signs of hypernatremia (e.g., thirst, agitation, and hyperreflexia), which indicates that too much fluid was removed or too much sodium was infused. Potassium loss may occur with diuretics as well, so the nurse should monitor for hypokalemia. **6**

Care must be taken in the use of hypertonic saline infusions to avoid rapid shifts in sodium level. The nurse should be aware of the length of time hyponatremia has been present and the severity of symptoms. If symptoms are severe and hyponatremia is acute over less than 48 hours, sodium supplement may be infused rapidly to avoid complications of the low sodium levels. Frequent sodium level determinations should reveal an increase of up to 2 mEq/L over 3–4 hours to a maximum of 15 mEq/day. If the sodium level has been low for more than 48 hours. **4**

- Infuse hypertonic saline (3% and 5% NaCl) slowly.

- Watch for signs of cerebral edema and neurologic disturbances, particularly if hyponatremia has been present for 48 hours or longer.

- Monitor serum sodium levels and report increases that exceed 0.5 mEq/h or 12 mEq/day.

If excessive ADH is present (SIADH), treatment usually involves

- Removal of the secreting tissue or tumor.

- Use of diuretics and fluid restriction as treatment, and the nurse should monitor for excessive treatment and dehydration, including intake and output, weight loss, and hypernatremia, as stated earlier.

- Supplements may be provided if a lack of aldosterone or cortisol is present. The nurse must monitor for signs of overtreatment, which would include signs of hypernatremia and of Cushing syndrome owing to excess cortisol. **6**

If infusion of sodium-free fluids resulted in hyponatremia, infusions are corrected by adding sodium. Diuretic therapy and sodium supplements may be used to restore balance. The precautions mentioned previously should be used.

Fluid and sodium supplements may be given if the decreased level of sodium is due to a loss through

- Vomiting
- Diarrhea
- Nasogastric tube drainage

The nurse should

- Monitor for fluid and sodium excess.
- Closely watch intake and output.
- Monitor weight.
- Monitor laboratory values for electrolytes.
- Monitor and treat blood glucose levels if fluid loss is due to hyperglycemia and osmotic diuresis to ensure that blood glucose levels are balanced.
- Monitor for hypoglycemia as a result of insulin therapy if indicated. **6**

The nurse should watch patients who are at risk for hyponatremia and implement care measures, including administering patient teaching to promote self-care when appropriate:

- Monitor patients with SIADH and teach patients with adrenal insufficiency that corticosteroids must be taken continuously (keep emergency doses in possession at all times).
- Instruct patients on the signs of adrenal crisis that may occur under physical (e.g., surgery or injury) or emotional stress:
  - Extreme weakness
  - Nausea and vomiting
  - Hypotension (may progress to shock)
  - Confusion
- Watch patients taking lithium for signs of toxicity when hyponatremia is present. This toxicity can occur even if the lithium dosage has been consistent because hyponatremia causes an increase in lithium retention.
- Instruct patients on lithium to maintain daily salt intake and watch for signs of lithium toxicity.

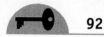

Caution these patients to maintain adequate salt intake, avoid or report periods of anorexia, and avoid diuretics or take them cautiously. These patients should be monitored frequently and will need to visit their primary-care providers regularly.

Conclusion

Sodium is the primary positive ion in extracellular fluid and is a major determinant of fluid concentration or extracellular osmolality. Sodium is present in the body in a variety of forms and is stored in the bones and, more prevalently, in body fluids. Sodium is important for blood pressure maintenance, nerve impulse conduction, and circulation of nutrients into the cell. Thus sodium imbalance (outside the 135–145 mEq/L range) can result in fluid imbalance, as well as other electrolyte imbalances.

Several additional key points should be noted from this chapter:

- Sodium concentration in the blood is regulated by absorption of sodium in the intestines and excretion of sodium through the kidneys.
- Aldosterone, ADH, and ANP control sodium and water retention or loss.
- Hypernatremia, an excess of sodium in the blood, can occur as a result of excess intake or decreased excretion.
- Fluid loss and dehydration are the most common causes of hypernatremia.
- Excess sodium accompanied by fluid excess can result in fluid retention, hypertension, and edema formation.
- Hyponatremia, an excessively low sodium level, can occur with excess diuretic usage, excess ADH or insufficient aldosterone (or cortisol) secretion, extreme perspiration (treated with salt-free fluids), vomiting, diarrhea, or nasogastric suctioning.
- Sodium imbalances can lead to other electrolyte imbalances, and if not corrected quickly, potassium imbalance can be fatal because imbalances can lead to nerve and cardiac dysfunction.
- Overtreatment of sodium imbalance could result in the opposite, sodium imbalance, as well as fluid and electrolyte (potassium) imbalances, if care is not exercised.

Case Application

Penny Parker, age 11, is admitted to the hospital after 4 days of nausea and vomiting, with only sips of water being retained. Penny is confused and combative.

Her skin is dry to the touch with dry mucous membranes. Her serum sodium level is 146 mEq/L (146 mmol/L). Vital signs show blood pressure (BP) 90/40 mm Hg, pulse (P) 120 beats/minute, respiration (R) 24 breaths/minute, and temperature (T) 37.2°C.

The nurse performs assessments to determine Penny's baseline status, establish needs, and anticipate interventions.

ASSESSMENTS: BASELINE AND NEEDS

- Penny is a child, so fluid loss has a more significant impact because the body fluid level is higher than in adults.
- Three days of vomiting with water for replacement likely will yield a hypovolemia and hemoconcentration, so the sodium level actually may be low once fluid volume is restored.
- Neurologic symptoms could be due to hypovolemia or electrolyte imbalance or a combination of both.
- Low blood pressure, tachypnea and tachycardia, and dry skin/membranes are likely the result of low blood volume and the body's attempt to circulate to tissues, but compensatory mechanism may be failing (blood pressure likely was higher initially).
- Temperature elevation is likely due to dehydration.
- Penny will need rehydration for hypovolemia that probably has been present for 72 hours or longer.

INTERVENTIONS

- Intravenous fluids—half-normal saline so that levels will not drop greatly, likely over 100 mL/h.
- Watch for symptoms of hypernatremia initially and hyponatremia after hydration.
- Sodium level determinations every 3 hours. Make sure that levels are not correcting too fast.
- Administer electrolytes every 6 hours. Note other electrolyte levels—potassium, calcium, etc.
- Monitor for signs of cerebral edema with fluid infusion—slow fluid and report.

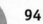

Final Check-up

1. A 25-year-old patient admitted after a car accident with head injury begins to have massive urine output (500 mL/h). The nurse is concerned that the patient will soon demonstrate a sodium imbalance. The nurse would anticipate which of the following treatment to address the sodium imbalance the patient is at highest risk for?

   (a) Increase intake of foods such as bananas.

   (b) Push 30–40 mL intravenous fluids hourly.

   (c) Administer aldactone (spiralactone).

   (d) Administer sodium supplements.

2. The nurse should watch which of the following patient most closely for hyponatremia?

   (a) Andy Peters, who eats canned vegetables three times each day

   (b) Aziz Akbar, who is a marathon runner and drinks water for hydration

   (c) Lola Ameriz, who has been constipated and is eating raw fruit for fiber

   (d) Bob Green, who exercises daily by swimming in an indoor pool

3. Bailey McIntosh, age 34, was in a motocycle accident. His arterial blood gases show a pH of 7.30, and the nurse infuses four times the standard amount of sodium bicarbonate as ordered. The nurse also infuses a normal saline drip at a rate of 200 mL/h. The nurse would watch closely for which of the following signs of a likely sodium imbalance?

   (a) Slow cardiac rhythm with a narrow QRS complex on electrocardiogram (ECG)

   (b) Increased respiratory rate with deep, regular breathing

   (c) Fluid buildup in extremities and pulmonary edema

   (d) Complaint of thirst and requests for large volumes of water

4. The nurse suspects that Mrs. Hong has a low sodium concentration. Which of the following pieces of information collected in the history would place Mrs. Hong at risk for hyponatremia?

   (a) A report of loose stools six to eight times per day for 4 days

   (b) A recent history of taking milk of magnesia for constipation

   (c) A past pregnancy resulting in aldosterone deficit

   (d) A recent episode of acute renal failure

5. Which of the following symptoms would indicate that the treatment for a patient with hypernatremia had been effective?

   (a) Patient's heart rate is 170 beats/miunte, and the rhythm is regular.

   (b) Patient's muscle tone and reflexes are hyporeactive.

   (c) Patient's lips and mucous membranes are moist.

   (d) Patient's urinary output is 20 mL or less per hour.

References

Needham A. *Comparative and Environmental Physiology: Acidosis and Alkalosis.* 2004.

Pagana KD, Pagana TJ. *Mosby's Manual of Diagnostic and Laboratory Tests,* 3rd ed. St. Louis: Mosby Elsevier, 2006.

Saladin K. *Anatomy and Physiology: The Unity of Form and Function,* 4th ed. New York: McGraw-Hill, 2007.

Web Site

http://en.wikipedia.org/wiki/Acidosis

CHAPTER 6

Potassium Imbalances: Hypokalemia and Hyperkalemia

Learning Objectives

At the end of this chapter, the student will be able to

1. Compare and contrast hypokalemia and hyperkalemia.

2. Identify patients at high risk for potassium imbalance.

3. Distinguish symptoms of excess and deficient potassium imbalances.

4. Identify diagnostic values associated with potassium imbalances.

5 Discuss the potential complications related to hypokalemia and hyperkalemia.

6 Determine the nursing implications related to treatments for potassium imbalances.

 Key Terms

Aldosterone	Hemolysis
Depolarization	Hypokalemia
Dialysate	Hyperkalemia
Dialysis	Hyperpolarization
Dysrhythmia	

Overview

Potassium, the major cation inside the cell, plays an important role in resting membrane potential and action potentials, affecting electrically excitable cells such as nerve and muscle cells. Most of the potassium in the body (98 percent) resides inside the cell, whereas the remaining 2 percent is in the extracellular fluid. Adequate amounts of potassium are obtained through daily ingestion. The daily requirement of potassium for the average adult is 40–50 mEq/day. Potassium is excreted through the kidneys (80 percent) and lost through the bowel (15 percent) and the sweat glands (5 percent).

The level of potassium in the cells and in the extracellular fluid will influence cell **depolarization**—the movement of the resting potential closer to the threshold at which an action potential can occur, causing more cell excitability and **hyperpolarization**—decreased resting membrane potential to a point far away from the threshold at which an action potential can occur, causing less cell excitability. Potassium imbalance thus can affect nerve and muscle cells by causing hyperexcitability or depressed excitability.

The most critical aspect of this electrolyte lies in the fact that potassium affects

- Muscle and nerve cells, which are key building blocks in heart tissue
- Cardiac rate, rhythm, and contractility, thus influencing cardiac output and tissue perfusion
- Muscle tissue function, including skeletal muscle and muscles of the diaphragm, which are required for breathing

- Nerve cells, which affect brain cells and tissue
- Regulation of many other body organs

Any deficit or excess in potassium levels can have a life-threatening effect on consciousness, mobility, and vitality.

The normal concentration of potassium in serum is in the range of 3.5–5.0 mEq/L (3.5–5.0 mmol/L). 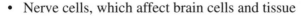 As stated in Chapters 1 and 3, potassium levels must be maintained within a narrow range to avoid the electrical disruptions that occur when the concentration of potassium is too high or too low. Potassium levels are regulated primarily through reabsorption and excretion in the kidneys.

A hormone produced in the adrenal gland, **aldosterone**, signals the kidneys to excrete or retain potassium based on the body's needs. If potassium levels are high, aldosterone is secreted, causing an increase in potassium excretion into the urine. Serum levels of potassium also are influenced by the levels of other electrolytes and acid–base balance. In alkalosis, for example, potassium may shift out of the cell as hydrogen ions shift into the cell to buffer the excessive acid, and when serum potassium concentration is low, potassium is retained by excreting sodium and chloride.

Drug therapy can alter potassium levels and should be noted to anticipate persons at risk or to identify possible sources of alterations when abnormal potassium levels are noted (Table 6–1).

Table 6–1   Drugs that Increase or Decrease Potassium Levels

Drugs that Increase Potassium Levels	**Drugs that Decrease Potassium Levels**
• Potassium-sparing diuretics • Potassium supplements • Antibiotics • Isoniazid (INH) • Lithium • Mannitol • Heparin • Epinephrine • Histamine • Antineoplastic drugs • Succinylcholine • Captopril	• Loop diuretics • Aspirin (acetylsalicylic acid or other salicylates) • Amphotericin B • Phenothiazines • Laxatives *Note:* The following may be used to reduce hyperkalemia: • Insulin and glucose • Bicarbonate (alkalosis) • Albuterol • Sodium polystyrene sulfonate (Kayexalate)

Hyperkalemia

Hyperkalemia is an excessively high level of potassium in the serum or plasma that involves a concentration of potassium ions greater than 5.0 mEq/L (5.0 mmol/L). It has been estimated that the body of a normal adult has about 3–6 mol of potassium ion. About 98 percent of this potassium is found inside various cells and organs, whereas only 0.4 percent is found in the serum. Hyperkalemia may be caused by an overall excess of body potassium or by a shift from inside to outside the cells. Under normal circumstances, the body has built-in mechanisms that prevent hyperkalemia owing to too much potassium intake in the diet.

- Certain cells and organs (e.g., kidneys) operate to prevent hyperkalemia by removing potassium from the blood after a meal.

- Another mechanism is vomiting. The intake of large amounts of potassium chloride induces the vomiting reflex, which helps to expel most of the potassium before it can be absorbed.

- A third way in which the body can eliminate excessive potassium ions is by way of the kidneys, which excrete potassium into the urine.

CAUSES AND SYMPTOMS 2 3 4

One of the most common cause of hyperkalemia is kidney (renal) disease. Additionally, potassium is released into the blood

- When cells are damaged, particularly in **hemolysis**—red blood cell (RBC) breakdown or destruction.
- With cell injury such as occurs owing to
  - Trauma or muscle destruction, including
    - Burns
    - Crush injuries
    - Conditions such as rhabdomyolysis
  - Rarely, strenuous exercise
- With the use of hemolytic drugs
- With infection

All these situations also can result in increased serum potassium levels. Because trauma and release of potassium from cells will elevate potassium levels, the nurse must take care that a false elevation of the level does not occur owing to tight tourniquet use or excessive hand clenching during specimen collection or that blood does not sit at room temperature for hours prior to delivery to the laboratory for testing. Other causes of hyperkalemia include

- Intake of too much of a potassium salt
- Infusion of old blood (owing to leakage of potassium from cells that have died)
- Acidosis (owing to the exchange of potassium for hydrogen ions in an attempt to restore acid–base balance)

Kidney damage will cause the glomerular filtration rate to be low and therefore result in hyperkalemia owing to decreased excretion of excess potassium, especially if high-potassium foods are consumed. The elderly are more prone to hyperkalemia because many of their regulatory functions tend to decline. Also, elderly patients who are being treated with certain drugs for high blood pressure that cause retention of potassium by the kidney are prone to hyperkalemia (Table 6–2).

Symptoms of hyperkalemia include rapid heart beat (fibrillation). In severe cases, the heart may stop beating (i.e., cardiac arrest). In less severe cases, the individual may develop nervous symptoms such as tingling of the skin, numbness of hands

Table 6–2   Factors that Increase Availability or Decrease Excretion of Potassium

Factors that Increase Potassium Availability	Factors that Decrease Potassium Excretion
• Excessive oral intake of potassium supplements • Excessive use of salt substitutes • Infusion of old blood • Rapid IV potassium infusion • Acidosis • Tissue damage owing to crush injury, burns, etc. • Chemotherapy (lysis of cells) Dehydration (hemoconcentrates potassium) *Note:* False elevation in lab values may occur owing to • Leukocytosis • Thrombocytosis • Hemolysis of specimen due to prolonged sitting • Excessive pressure on extremity during blood draw (tourniquet, hand clenching)	• Renal failure • Potassium-sparing diuretics • Hypoaldosteronism

and feet, weakness, or a flaccid paralysis that is characteristic of both hyperkalemia and hypokalemia. **1**

NURSING IMPLICATIONS IN THE TREATMENT OF HYPERKALEMIA **6**

Treatment of the underlying cause is ideal, when possible. Renal failure, the major cause of hyperkalemia, cannot be fully resolved (unless it is an acute, temporary renal failure). The failed renal functioning is addressed by **dialysis**—the cleansing of the blood using an artificial kidney or using the peritoneal cavity to filter waste products, excess electrolytes, and fluid. The nurse must monitor the patient's vital signs and laboratory values carefully during the dialysis process for early detection of excessive removal of fluids and changes in electrolytes. The speed of dialysis or concentration of **dialysate**—the fluid used to establish a concentration exchange gradient—may need to be adjusted to obtain the desired fluid and electrolyte levels.

If trauma or damaged tissues are the cause of the hyperkalemia, actions to prevent further tissue damage, such as antibiotics and bed rest, will reduce cell death and the release of potassium. The expiration dates on blood products should be monitored carefully, and the nurse should stop any infusion of blood if a rise in potassium level is noted.

If the acidosis causing the hyperkalemia is extreme, bicarbonate may be administered to restore acid–base balance. If other electrolyte imbalances are noted, the appropriate treatment (e.g., chloride replacement) should be implemented. Care should be taken when providing supplements for electrolyte replacement. Electrolyte and acid–base levels should be monitored carefully to prevent overtreatment and additional electrolyte imbalance or alkalosis.

SPEED BUMP

1. Which of the following pieces of clinical information indicates that the patient is at risk for hyperkalemia?

(a) There are frequent premature ventricular contractions.

(b) Arterial blood gases reveal a pH above 7.50.

(c) There is a burn injury over 40 percent of the patient's body.

(d) Renal calculi are seen owing to hypercalcemia from protein release of Ca^+.

2. Which of the following pieces of information from the patient's history would alert the nurse to watch the patient closely for signs of hyperkalemia?

(a) The patient was diagnosed with chronic renal failure 6 years ago.

(b) The patient is taking furosemide (Lasix) three times a day.

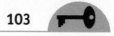

(c) The dietary history reveals a high intake of nuts and melons.

(d) The occupation history indicates work outside in intense heat.

3. The nurse would monitor for which of the following signs that the treatment provided to a patient for hyperkalemia may be excessive?

(a) The patient is alert and oriented to person, place, and time.

(b) The nurse hears rales in the patient's lung fields.

(c) The patient's urine output remains 10 mL/h for 3 hours.

(d) The patient demonstrates an irregular cardiac rhythm.

Hypokalemia

Hypokalemia is an abnormally low potassium level in the serum. As stated earlier, potassium is necessary for nerve cell conduction and contraction of muscles, including the heart. It is also needed for proper enzyme activity, and it facilitates cell membrane function. In hypokalemia, the adrenal gland retains the hormone aldosterone, and the kidneys conserve potassium when more is needed. A proper balance of potassium is needed for normal health, and the normal range of potassium concentration is 3.5–5.0 mEq/L. If the potassium level falls below 3.5 mEq/L, then one may suffer from hypokalemia. **4**

CAUSES AND SYMPTOMS

The two major causes of hypokalemia are

- Excretion of the body's potassium
- Excessive uptake of potassium by muscles from fluids in the immediate environment

One of the most common causes of hypokalemia is the use of diuretic drugs. Diuretics are used for many different medical conditions, and this accounts for the high percent of hypokalemia in the elderly. These drugs increase the excretion of water and salts in the urine. Other causes of hypokalemia include

- Excessive perspiration/sweating
- Vomiting
- Diarrhea
- Fasting

- Starvation
- Magnesium deficiency
- Alkalosis

Since potassium is needed to control muscle action, hypokalemia can cause the heart to stop beating. Young infants are especially at risk from this cause, especially when severe diarrhea continues for a week or longer. Vomiting causes an increase in potassium loss in urine. In most people after 3 weeks of fasting, the potassium level in the blood will decline to below 3.0 mEq/L, which results in severe hypokalemia

Symptoms vary depending on whether the condition is mild or severe. In mild cases, no symptoms may occur. Moderate cases may result in

- Disorientation
- Confusion
- Discomfort of muscles
- Muscle weakness

Severe hypokalemia results in

- Extreme weakness of the body
- Occasional paralysis
- Paralysis of the muscles of the lung, resulting in death

In very severe cases, hypokalemia can cause abnormal heart beat (i.e., **dysrhythmia**) that can lead to death from cardiac arrest. Hypokalemia also can result in hypochloremia as the body attempts to retain potassium by excreting sodium and chloride.

NURSING IMPLICATIONS IN TREATMENT OF HYPOKALEMIA 6

Treatment of the underlying problem is critical to resolution of hypokalemia. If diuretic use is involved, a different diuretic that is potassium-sparing may be chosen. If perspiration, vomiting, or diarrhea is the cause of the hypokalemia, the condition (i.e., infection or toxin) causing the sweating, vomiting, or diarrhea is treated with antibiotics or antitoxins. Fasting or starvation is addressed by dietary intake or parenteral nutrition sufficient to prevent muscle breakdown for energy. If magnesium deficiency is the cause of the diuresis resulting in potassium loss, magnesium supplements may be provided to restore balance. Excessive supplementation could cause magnesium excess. Table 6–3 lists some foods that have a high potassium content.

Table 6–3   Foods with High Content of Potassium

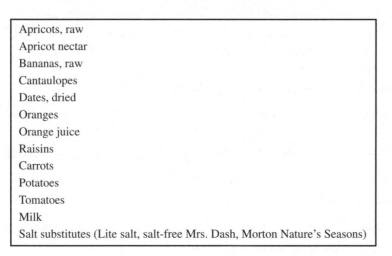

Apricots, raw
Apricot nectar
Bananas, raw
Cantaulopes
Dates, dried
Oranges
Orange juice
Raisins
Carrots
Potatoes
Tomatoes
Milk
Salt substitutes (Lite salt, salt-free Mrs. Dash, Morton Nature's Seasons)

Regardless of the cause of the hypokalemia, potassium supplements usually are provided to diminish the symptoms and complications. Caution is taken with potassium supplements to avoid excess. If hypokalemia is caused by alkalosis, particular caution is taken with supplements because the correction of alkalosis will cause potassium to shift back out of the cells, and supplements could result in a potassium excess.

Case Application

Mr. Lawrence Key, age 62, was admitted 5 days ago after a car accident with massive injuries to his extremities and trunk. Vital signs are blood pressure (BP) 100/60 mm Hg, pulse (P) 118 beats/minute, and respiration (R) 32 breaths/minute. He is lethargic, his skin is cool to the touch, and his mucous membranes are dry. His laboratory a results today revealed Na^+ 137 mEq/L, K^+ 4.9 mEq/L, CO_2 20 mEq/L, blood urea nitrogen (BUN) 40 mg/dL, and creatinine 2.7 mg/dL. His urine output has been 20 mL/h except when a diuretic (Lasix) was administered. The nurse considers the following when analyzing Mr. Key's risk for potassium imbalance:

- Mr. Key's age places him at risk because of decreased renal function accompanying aging.

- The massive trauma resulted several conditions that increase potassium concentration:

- Cell injury caused the release of potassium from cells.
- Circulatory compromise (i.e., decreased level of consciousness, low BP, tachycardia, cool skin, and dry mucous membranes indicate possible shock) decreases renal perfusion and excretion of K^+, resulting in hyperkalemia.
- K^+ level is elevated, indicating hyperkalemia.
- CO_2 is low, indicating low bicarbonate and possible acidosis pulling potassium out of the cells and driving H^+ ions into the cells.
- BUN and creatinine are elevated, indicating renal insufficiency/failure.

The nurse should explore Mr. Key's history and other data to analyze additional risk factors, including

- History of chronic illnesses (e.g., Addison's is disease or hypoaldosteronism)
- Medications being taken (see Table 6–1)
- Previous renal condition
- Prior hydration status (potassium is increased in dehydration)
- Electrocardiogram (ECG)—note dysrhythmia secondary to high potassium levels
- Muscle weakness
- Neurostatus (i.e., tingling and other changes may be difficult to assess while altered, but further decrease in sensorium should be noted)

The nurse might anticipate the therapy to control the potassium levels:

- Diuretics to promote renal function and cause potassium excretion
- Glucose and insulin if potassium level becomes severely elevated
- Kayexalate or other drugs as needed to reduce potassium
- Monitor for hypokalemia owing to therapy
- Monitor laboratory values frequently
- Monitor renal function (if diuresis occurs, hypokalemia may result)

Conclusion

Potassium is the primary positive ion inside the cell and is essential for normal cell function. Potassium plays a vital role in electrical impulse generation and thus has a critical role in muscle and nerve function. The major impact of a potassium deficit or excess is in the regulation of cardiac rhythm and the function of the muscles, including cardiac muscle. Additionally, potassium imbalance (outside the 3.5–5.0 mEq/L range) can result in other electrolyte imbalances and acid–base imbalances, and acid–base and electrolyte imbalances, in turn, can cause potassium imbalance.

Several additional key points should be noted from this chapter:

- Hyperkalemia, an excess level of potassium in the blood, can occur as a result of excess intake, decreased excretion, or movement of potassium from inside the cells to the extracellular fluid.

- A rapid increase in potassium resulting in excess can result in cells becoming hyperexcitable, leading to cardiac arrest, whereas a slow rise in potassium to excessive levels will cause a depression of action potentials and neuromuscular reactivity.

- Renal failure is a major cause of hyperkalemia.

- Addison's disease, burns, injuries to muscles, and other tissues; potassium-sparing drugs; and acidosis also can lead to hyperkalemia.

- Hypokalemia, an excessively low potassium level, can occur with excess diuretic usage, excess aldosterone secretion, perspiration, vomiting, diarrhea, fasting, and starvation.

- Potassium imbalances can lead to acid–base and other electrolyte imbalances, and if not corrected quickly, potassium imbalance can be fatal because imbalances can lead to nerve and cardiac dysfunction.

- Overtreatment of one potassium imbalance could result in the opposite potassium imbalance if care is not exercised.

Final Check-up

1. A 55-year-told patient was admitted after a car accident with crush injury to the chest and extremities. The nurse is concerned that the patient is demonstrating a potassium imbalance. The nurse would anticipate which of the following treatments to address the potassium imbalance for which the patient is at the highest risk?

   (a) Increase intake of foods such as bananas.

   (b) Push 50–100 mL of intravenous fluids hourly.

   (c) Administer aldactone (spiralactone).

   (d) Administer potassium supplements.

2. The nurse should watch which of the following patients most closely for hypokalemia?

   (a) Andy Peters, who eats three to four bananas daily

   (b) Aziz Akbar, who has acute renal failure

   (c) Lola Ameriz, who had diarrhea for 3 days

   (d) Bob Brown, who exercises strenuously daily

3. Bailey McIntosh has had 300–400 mL of urine each hour over the past 26 hours. The nurse would watch closely for which of the following signs of a likely potassium imbalance?

   (a) Slow cardiac rhythm with a wide QRS complex on ECG

   (b) Increased respiratory rate with deep, regular breathing

   (c) Fluid buildup in the extremities and pulmonary edema

   (d) Complaint of thirst and requests for large volumes of water

4. The nurse suspects that Mrs. Hong has a low potassium concentration. Which of the following pieces of information collected in the history would place Mrs. Hong at risk for hypokalemia?

   (a) A report of loose stools six to eight times per day for 4 days

   (b) A recent history of taking milk of magnesia for constipation

   (c) A past pregnancy resulting in an aldosterone deficit

   (d) A recent episode of acute renal failure

5. Which of the following symptoms indicate a complication that is likely to occur with hypokalemia?

   (a) Increased bowel activity with diarrhea

   (b) Decreased cardiac

   (c) Increased irritability—disorientation and confusion

   (d) Decreased renal output and edema formation

6. Which of the following symptoms would indicate that the treatment for a patient with hypokalemia had been effective?

   (a) Patient's heart rate is 70 beats/minute, and rhythm is regular.

   (b) Patient's muscle tone and reflexes are hyporeactive.

   (c) Patient's respiratory rate is 36 breaths/minute and shallow.

   (d) Patient's urinary output is 100 mL/h or greater.

7. Which of the following questions would provide the most important data to support the nurse's concern that a patient was hyperkalemic?

   (a) Has the patient eaten large portions of red meat or fruit recently?

   (b) Does the patient have a sedentary lifestyle?

   (c) Has the patient experienced muscle cramps recently?

   (d) Does the patient smoke more than two packs of cigarettes daily?

References

Metheny NM. *Fluid and Electrolyte Balance: Nursing Considerations,* 4th ed. Philadelphia: Lippincott, 2000.

Needham A. *Comparative and Environmental Physiology Acidosis and Alkalosis.* 2004

Pagana KD, Pagana TJ. *Mosby's Manual of Diagnostic and Laboratory Tests,* 3rd ed. St. Louis: Mosby Elsevier, 2006.

Saladin K. *Anatomy and Physiology: The Unity of Form and Function,* 4th ed. New York: McGraw-Hill, 2007.

Web Site

http://en.wikipedia.org/wiki/Acidosis

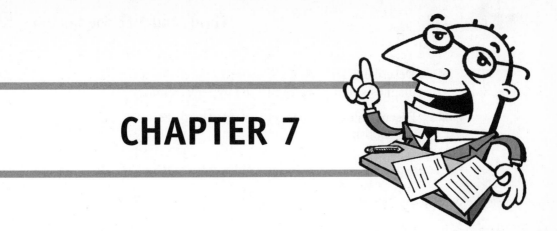

CHAPTER 7

Calcium Imbalances: Hypocalcemia and Hypercalcemia

Learning Objectives

At the end of this chapter, the student will be able to

1. Describe the process of normal calcium metabolism in the human body.

2. State the normal value range for total serum calcium and ionized calcium.

3. Compare and contrast causes, manifestations, and treatments for hypocalcemia and hypercalcemia.

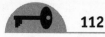

4 Describe diagnostic tests and procedures that are used in making a definitive diagnosis of hypocalcemia and hypercalcemia.

5 Discuss nursing intervention related to the treatment of impaired calcium metabolism.

🔑 Key Terms

Extravasation	Osteomalacia
Hypocalcemia	Osteoporosis
Hypercalcemia	Rickets
Hypoparathyroidism	Tetany
Hyperphosphatemia	

Overview

Calcium is the most abundant mineral in the human body. It is found predominantly in the bones and teeth, which act as a storage reserve for serum calcium. In fact, 99 percent of the body's calcium is stored in the bones and teeth. The remaining 1 percent is found in the bloodstream in two forms, ionized or bound to protein. Calcium plays a critical role in building and maintaining strong bones and teeth. Additionally, calcium is important for several other physiologic processes, including normal cell function, neural transmission, muscle contractility, wound healing, and intracellular signaling.

1 Under normal circumstances, the body maintains the required balance between the calcium found in the tissues and the calcium obtained in the diet. The normal value range for total serum calcium varies with the age of the individual. The normal range for adults is 8.6–10.3 mg/dL (2.23–2.57 mmol/L). In certain situations, ionized calcium levels, which in adults should be between 4.65 and 5.28 mg/dL (1.03 and 1.23 mmol/L), provide a better picture of whether or not adequate calcium is present. This is particularly true when a protein deficiency exist because 50 percent of the calcium found in the body is bound to protein. Proper functioning of the parathyroid gland, adequate levels of vitamin D, and normal kidney function also affect calcium levels. An imbalance in calcium metabolism results in either **hypocalcemia** (calcium levels below 8.6 mg/dL) or **hypercalcemia** (calcium levels above 10.0 mg/dL). **2**

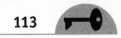

Hypocalcemia

CAUSES AND SYMPTOMS

Hypocalcemia can be caused by a number of factors, including, but not limited to,

- Inadequate intake of dietary calcium
- Malabsorption of calcium from the intestinal tract
- Vitamin D deficiency
- **Hyperphosphatemia**
- **Hypoparathyroidism**

Inadequate intake of dietary calcium is caused most often by a lack of the right food sources of this nutrient in the diet. Dairy products are the most abundant source of calcium, but there are other good sources of calcium. This is particularly important for lactose-intolerant individuals to know in order to avoid hypocalcemia. **3**

Development Considerations

- Newborns, especially premature or small for gestational age babies, may develop neonatal hypocalcemia related to an immature parathyroid gland.
- The infant may or may not have any symptoms.
- Treatment may or may not be required. If required, treatment includes calcium supplement either by mouth or intravenously.

Vitamin D is important in calcium absorption. While milk and some other foods are fortified with vitamin D and may provide a good source of this nutrient, the most important source of vitamin D is exposure to sunlight. Absorption of calcium is just as important in the prevention of hypocalcemia as is adequate dietary intake. Calcium is absorbed primarily from the small intestines. Thus disorders causing malabsorption in the small intestines, particularly the duodenum, should be considered in determining underlying causes of hypocalcemia. Alcoholism or disorders that prevent absorption of fats also can cause hypocalcemia because, as mentioned previously, 50 percent of calcium is bound to protein. Furthermore, foods high in phytic acid (e.g., spinach, sweet potatoes, and beans) and oxalic acids (e.g., whole-grain breads, seeds, and nuts) may bind to calcium and prevent its optimal absorption. Hyperphosphatemia, which may occur as a result of too many laxatives and enemas that have high phosphate levels, can cause hypocalcemia as well.

REGULATION

When the calcium concentration drops below normal, the parathyroid gland secretes parathyroid hormone (PTH). This hormone stimulates bone-reabsorbing cells (i.e., osteocytes and osteoblasts), which cause an increase in calcium and phosphate ions in the extracellular fluid. PTH in association with vitamin D also can stimulate the absorption of calcium indirectly from the intestine and cause the kidney to conserve calcium ions and excrete phosphate ions. Therefore, any damage to the parathyroid gland or the kidneys or failure of the body to produce 1,25-dihydroxy vitamin D will prevent mobilization of calcium from the bones and intestine to the blood plasma. This will lead to hypocalcemia. **1** **3**

Symptoms of hypocalcemia vary depending on the severity and duration of the deficiency, and in some cases, a patient even may be asymptomatic. If a patient is symptomatic, initial complaints may include numbness and/or tingling around the mouth or in the hands and feet; muscles spasms in the feet, face, and hands that in more severe cases may expand to **tetany** (uncontrolled muscle contraction): seizures, bronchospasms accompanied by respiratory distress, and cardiac arrhythmias. Low levels of calcium in the bones may lead to disorders such as decreased bone minereralization referred to as **rickets** in children, **osteomalacia** in adults, or **osteoporosis** (a condition more prominent in postmenopausal women).

There is no single test or procedure available for making a definitive diagnosis of hypocalcemia. Instead, diagnosis should be based on the history, presenting signs and symptoms, and laboratory and procedure results. The laboratory diagnostic workup may include calcium, phosphorous, magnesium, albumin, vitamin D, and parathyroid hormone tests. Tests or procedures to evaluate kidney function, liver function, and bone density also may be beneficial. It is important that test results are accurate and reflect actual levels in the body. **4**

Passing the Test

Affect laboratory result accuracy

- Nutritional supplements
- Antacids
- Vitamin D
- Thiazide diuretics
- Lithium
- Thyroxine

(continued)

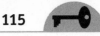

Supplemental laboratory tests

- Phosphorous
- Vitamin D
- Parathyroid hormone (PTH)
- Magnesium
- Albumin
- Comprehensive metabolic panel

Other test

- Bone density scan

NURSING IMPLICATIONS

Treatment of hypocalcemia varies and is directed toward correcting the underlying causes. Initial nursing interventions will depend primarily on the condition of the patient at the time he or she presents for treatment. Nursing interventions focus on stabilizing the patient who presents with life-threatening manifestations such as

- Respiratory distress
- Tetany
- Cardiac arrhythmias

Intravenous (IV) administration of calcium may be required to stabilize the patient and should be administered cautiously and at the prescribed rate to avoid cardiac complications. The IV site should be monitored closely because some calcium compounds may cause severe tissue damage if **extravasation** (leakage into tissues) occurs. A thiazide diuretic may be ordered to facilitate reabsorption of calcium from the kidneys. If this is the case, the patient's weight, intake, and output must be monitored.

Once the patient is stabilized, or if the patient is stable at the time of presentation, initial efforts will be directed toward assisting with determining the underlying cause of the hypocalcemia. The nurse will interview the patient to ascertain dietary habits and discuss the importance of intake of a variety of sources of calcium and vitamin D. **5**

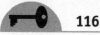

5 Tips: Keeping Your Calcium at the Right Speed

- Diary products are a great source of calcium.

- Suggest green leafy vegetables to individuals who are lactose tintolerant.

- Some otherwise healthy foods interfere with calcium absorption (those high in phytic acid and oxalic acid).

- Get plenty of sunlight (best method of vitamin D synthesis).

- Do not smoke (may increase bone loss).

- Use laxatives cautiously

The nurse also should discuss lifestyle practices (e.g., living environment, use of recreational drugs and alcohol, etc.). An inquiry should be made about the presence of such related conditions such as

- Pancreatitis
- Gastrointestinal disorders
- Liver disorders
- Kidney disorders
- Fractures
- Itchy dry skin
- Numbness
- Tingling sensations
- Recent surgeries

A thorough assessment of physical and behavioral signs also should be included. Specifically, the nurse should observe for the presence of twitching, tremors, dry skin, course hair, tooth decay, and alterations in mental status.

A mainstay in nursing interventions for patients with hypocalcemia is education: **5**

- Dietary sources of calcium should be reviewed with the patient.
- Consideration should be given to the patient's dietary preferences and to intolerances that the patient may have.
- The nurse also should ensure that the patient knows how to read food labels.
- In some cases, a dietary supplement of calcium may be recommended for the patient.

- The nurse should ensure that the patient knows how to take the medication properly.
- The patient should understand that no more than 500 mg of calcium should be consumed at one time. Taking more will not provide any added benefit because the body can absorb only up to the 500 mg at one time.
- It is also important that the patient understand the dangers of overmedicating himself or herself.
- Dietary sources of calcium should remain a part of the patient's diet even if he or she is taking a calcium supplement. The patient also should have an adequate intake of vitamin D and magnesium.
- The role sunlight exposure plays in vitamin D production should be discussed with the patient.
- The nurse always must keep in mind that the success of educating the patient rests heavily on the patient's active participation in development and acceptance of the plan.

SPEED BUMP

1. *Which of the following would best counter the occurrence of hypocalcemia?*
   (a) Exposure to sunlight on a regular basis
   (b) Inclusion of foods such as spinach, nuts, and whole-grain breads in the diet
   (c) Supplementing the diet with 1000 mg of calcium daily
   (d) Supplementing the diet with 1000 mg of phosphorous daily

2. *Which of the following findings would lead the nurse to suspect hypophosphatemia as a possible underlying cause of a patient's hypercalcemia?*
   (a) Ionic calcium level below 4.65 mg/dL
   (b) Patient's report of experiencing tingling sensations around the mouth
   (c) Patient's report of using laxatives on a regular basis
   (d) Presence of albumin in the urine

3. *Which of the following interventions is most appropriate for a hospitalized patient who has been admitted to stabilize severe hypocalcemia?*
   (a) Administer loop diuretics as prescribe by the physician.
   (b) Closely monitor the patient's heart rate and rhythm.
   (c) Closely monitor the patient's deep tendon reflexes.
   (d) Place the patient in soft restraints to avoid injury.

Hypercalcemia

CAUSES AND SYMPTOMS

Hypercalcemia is an abnormal increase in blood calcium, usually more than 10.5 mg/dL. Many different conditions can cause hypercalcemia; the most common are hyperparathyroidism and cancer. Hypercalcemia is the most common life-threatening metabolic disorder associated with neoplastic disease, occurring in an estimated 10–20 percent of all adults with cancer. Cancers of the lung, breast, kidney, neck, and head, as well as certain hematologic malignancies (e.g., multiple myeloma), often are accompanied by hypercalcemia. With certain types of cancer, a protein is produced that mimics PTH, which, in turn, stimulates the release of calcium from the bones into the blood, thus contributing to hypercalcemia. In other instances, the effects of the cancer are related to the consequences of the disease, such as immobility, vomiting, and dehydration. Immobility counters weight bearing by the bones, resulting in the release of calcium from the bones into the bloodstream. Vomiting and dehydration decrease the excretion of calcium by the kidneys. Long-term excessive intake of calcium or vitamin D supplements also may contribute to the occurrence of hypercalcemia.

Few patients experience all the symptoms that have been associated with hypercalcemia, and some patients may not experience any at all. Some patients develop signs and symptoms when calcium is only slightly elevated, whereas others with long-standing hypercalcemia may tolerate serum calcium levels higher than 13 mg/dL with few symptoms. Common symptoms of hypercalcemia include loss of appetite, nausea, vomiting, constipation, and abdominal pain. Hypercalcemia causes a reversible tubular defect in the kidney, resulting in loss of the ability to concentrate urine and subsequent polyuria. Decreased fluid intake and polyuria lead to dehydration, which is manifested by the presence of thirst, dry mucosae, and diminished or absence of sweating. Symptoms become more serious as calcium levels rise. Kidney stones may form, and waste products can build up. Muscles may become weak, blood plasma rises, and heart rhythm may change. Loss of bone mass is also a concern. Other symptoms include mood swings, confusion, and in severe cases, coma and death. **1 3**

NURSING IMPLICATIONS

Severe cases of hypercalcemia may require hospitalization, in which case the patient is likely to receive IV fluids for rehydration and administration of medications that counter bone breakdown. Loop diuretics such as furosemide (Lasix) may be administered to increase the excretion of calcium from the kidneys.

Other medications that may be prescribed include calcitonin to slow bone loss and glucocorticoids to counter excessive amounts of vitamin D in the blood. If there is kidney impairment, hemodialysis also may be required to remove excess waste and calcium. Supportive nursing care of the hospitalized patient includes monitoring intake and output, promoting comfort, and preventing stress or strain on the bones when moving the patient. Providing emotional support for the patient, significant others, and family members is also a central theme in the care of these patients. **5**

The physician may recommend surgical removal of the parathyroid glands for patients who have been diagnosed with primary hyperparathyroidism. Surgery usually is preceded by the administration of a small dose of radioactive material to locate the diseased gland(s). A small approximately 1-in incision is made in the neck under local anesthesia. In most cases the patient is discharged home a few hours after surgery. Routine nursing care is no different from that provided for any preoperative outpatient surgery. The patient is screened for possible contraindications, laboratory test results are reviewed, consent is obtained, and emotional support is provided. During the postoperative phase, the patient's vital signs are monitored closely, a safe environment is provided to prevent injury, and discharge instructions related to care during the immediate recuperative phase are given to the patient, significant other, and/or family member accompanying the patient. Possible risks associated with surgical removal of the parathyroid glands include damage to the nerves that control the vocal cords and the development of chronically low levels of calcium. **5**

As with hypocalcemia, patient education related to self-care is important. The patient should be instructed to drink plenty of fluids, take only the medications prescribed by the physician, refrain from smoking, and exercise once cleared to do so by the physician. Both strength training and weight-bearing exercises are recommended. The patient should increase the time and duration of exercise sessions gradually. **5**

---

3 Hypocalcemia

- Numbness and tingling
- Muscle spasms
- Tetany
- Seizures
- Bronchospasms
- Cardiac arrhythmias*

Hypercalcemia

- Loss of appetite
- Nausea/vomiting
- Constipation
- Abdominal pain
- Polyuria
- Dehydration

(continued)

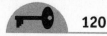

- Cataracts
- Rickets (children)
- Osteomalacia (adults)
- Osteoporosis (postmenopausal)
- Changes in mental status*

*Both hypocalcemia and hypercalcemia

- Kidney stones
- Muscle weakness
- Cardiac arrhythmias*
- Changes in mental status*

Conclusion

Key points in this chapter include

- Calcium plays a critical role in the proper functioning of several physiologic processes in the human body, most notably healthy bones and teeth.
- Under normal circumstances, the body is efficient at maintaining the required balance among the intake, absorption, storage, and excretion of calcium.
- Disturbances in this delicate balance may be related to dietary imbalances, environmental influences, disorders of absorption, and/or organ dysfunction.
- A patient may be asymptomatic; exhibit mild manifestations such as numbness, tingling, and spasms; or may experience life-threatening conditions (e.g., respiratory distress, cardiac arrhythmias, and tetany).
- It is imperative that consideration be given to multiple variables when attempting to determine the specific calcium imbalance and the underlying cause.
- Appropriate treatment can be initiated only if proper identification of the cause of the calcium imbalance occurs.

Final Check-up

1. What percentage of serum calcium is bound to protein?
   (a) 1 percent
   (b) 10 percent
   (c) 50 percent
   (d) 99 percent

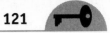

2. Which of the following findings would the nurse consider to be significant for a patient who is suspected of having hypercalcemia?

   (a) Diarrhea

   (b) Excessive intake of phosphorous

   (c) Polyuria

   (d) Profuse sweating

3. A 60-year-old woman is admitted to the hospital for treatment of hypercalcemia. During the medication reconciliation process, the patient states that she is taking the medications listed below. Which one of these medications is most significant to the patient's diagnosis of hypercalcemia?

   (a) Estrogen

   (b) Laxative

   (c) Potassium supplement

   (d) Thiazide diuretic

4. Which of the following underlying disorders places the patient at the greatest risk for developing hypercalcemia?

   (a) Hyperparathyroidism

   (b) Myxedema

   (c) Osteoporosis

   (d) Ovarian cancer

5. A definitive diagnosis of hypercalcemia should be based on which of the following diagnostic tests?

   (a) Bone density scan

   (b) Ionized calcium test

   (c) Total serum calcium test

   (d) None of the above

6. Which of the following patients is at greatest risk for developing osteomalacia?

   (a) A 5-year-old homeless child whose primary food source is rice

   (b) A 36-year-old bed-ridden patient who also has lactose intolerance

   (c) A 42-year-old who spends 3–4 hours outside daily

   (d) A 50-year-old postmenopausal female

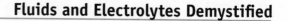
7. The nurse is providing preoperative teaching to a patient who is scheduled to have surgery to remove diseased parathyroid gland(s). Which of the following preoperative instructions would be *incorrect*?

   (a) An approximately 1-in incision will be made in your neck.

   (b) A small amount of radioactive material will be administered prior to the procedure.

   (c) Your hospital stay will be approximately 3 days.

   (d) Lifelong calcium and vitamin D supplements may be required after surgery.

8. Which self-care instructions should be given to a patient who has a diagnosis of hypercalcemia?

   (a) Avoid weight-bearing exercises.

   (b) Avoid strength training exercises.

   (c) Limit fluid intake as prescribed by the doctor.

   (d) Refrain from smoking.

Reference

Postgraduate Medicine 2005;118:49–50.

Web Sites

www.nlm.nih.gov/medlineplus/ency/article/000365.htm
www.nlm.nih.gov/medlineplus/print/ency/article/003477.htm
www.labtestsonline.org/understanding/analytes/calcium/glance.html
www.emedicine.com/emerg/topic271.htm
www.mayoclinic.com/print/hypercalcemia/DS00976/DSECTION=all&METHOD=print

CHAPTER 8

Magnesium Imbalances: Hypomagnesemia and Hypermagnesemia

Learning Objectives

At the end of this chapter, the student will be able to

1. Compare and contrast hypomagnesemia and hypermagnesemia.
2. Identify individuals at high risk for magnesium imbalance.
3. Distinguish symptoms of excess and deficient magnesium levels.
4. Identify diagnostic values associated with magnesium imbalances.

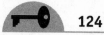

5 Discuss the potential complications related to hypomagnesemia and hypermagnesemia.

6 Determine the nursing implications related to treatments for magnesium imbalances.

Key Terms

Eclampsia/toxemia of pregnancy   Hypomagnesemia

Hemodialysis   Hypermagnesemia

Overview

Magnesium is the fourth most abundant cation in the body and the second most abundant cation within the cell (intracellularly). Magnesium is an important cation needed in cellular function, including protein and nucleic acid synthesis. Magnesium is critical for over 300 biochemical reactions in the body, including neuromuscular function and blood coagulation. Magnesium is very important in many biologic reactions that provide energy for cellular processes. It is responsible for the formation of adenosine triphosphate (ATP) in the mitochondria and the reverse reaction that breaks down ATP to adenosine diphosphate (ADP). Additionally, magnesium is needed for healthy bones, teeth, nerves, and muscles. It also prevents osteoporosis, decreases the risk of heart attack and strokes, and helps to prevent cardiovascular diseases and irregular heartbeats.

Magnesium acts on the myoneural junction and affects neuromuscular excitability. The reference range for the serum concentration of magnesium is 1.3–2.5 mEq/L (0.65–1.25 mmol/L). Concentrations above (i.e., **hypermagnesemia**) or below (i.e., **hypomagnesemia**) these levels can lead to imbalances. As magnesium levels increase, neuromuscular function is depressed, whereas a deficient level of magnesium results in increased excitability. **1** Magnesium homeostasis involves the kidney, small intestine, and bones, and imbalances usually are observed in hospital populations (patient illnesses).

Magnesium is found in all cells and makes up about 0.05 percent of body weight. Approximately 50 percent is deposited in the bones as phosphates or carbonates. The remainder is found in tissues, of which 1–2 percent is in the extracellular fluid.

- Magnesium is located inside the cells (50 percent).
- Magnesium also is located in bone (48–49 percent) bound with phosphate.
- Magnesium also is located in blood plasma (1–2 percent).

Magnesium contributes to stable bone structure and the absorption and metabolism of calcium, as well as parathyroid hormone (PTH), a calcium-regulating hormone. In addition, magnesium contributes to carbohydrate metabolism. Studies have shown that a high intake of magnesium, calcium, and potassium, with low intake of sodium and fats, has a positive impact on hypertension. Additionally, magnesium deficit may contribute to heart attacks, dysrhythmias, and stroke. Magnesium sulfate may be used as a laxative, acting by osmotic retention of fluid, which increases the fluid in feces, distends the colon, and stimulates evacuation of feces. Magnesium sulfate may be used as a mechanism for bowel cleansing prior to surgery or an endoscopic procedure.

Magnesium levels are regulated by gastrointestinal absorption and renal excretion and reabsorption. Daily dietary intake usually provides a common source of magnesium. It can be obtained from nuts, green vegetables, wheat, coca products (chocolates), chlorophyll, meats, and seafood. Less than 40 percent of dietary magnesium is absorbed. However, most of the absorption takes place in the small intestine (mainly in the ileum). A smaller percentage of magnesium is also absorbed in the colon (sigmoid) and the rectum. As protein intake increases, absorption usually increases. Conversely, magnesium absorption decreases as calcium and vitamin D intake increases. Magnesium therefore is important in maintaining normal calcium concentrations in the blood.

Hypernatremia and hypercalcemia can result in decreased magnesium reabsorption. Magnesium may contribute to hypokalemia and associated symptoms. Symptoms of magnesium imbalance occasionally will be mixed with symptoms of calcium or potassium imbalance.

The recommended daily allowance (RDA) for magnesium is 4.5 mg/kg per day for adults. It is higher during pregnancy and lactation and also increases for individuals of a high-fat diet or taking high amounts of calcium and potassium. Magnesium reserves are stored in bones, some in the kidneys, and excess is excreted in the urine.

Hypermagnesemia

Hypermagnesemia, a rare condition, is an elevation of the serum magnesium level higher than 2.5 mEq/L (1.25 mmol/L). Since the kidneys are very effective in excreting excess magnesium, hypermagnesemia occurs very rarely. Therefore, the most common occurrences of hypermagnesemia would be in patients whose kidneys cannot excrete magnesium in sufficient quantities to maintain magnesium homeostasis. Hypermagnesemia also has been reported after taking enemas containing magnesium salts. This condition is sometimes seen in healthy patients who take excessive amounts of laxatives, pain relievers, and magnesium-containing antacids. ⬤

Because magnesium is an electrolyte that helps with nerve and muscle function, excessive concentrations of magnesium can severely disrupt body function. As magnesium levels increase, reflexes are lost and progress from loss of deep tendon reflexes to sleepiness and ultimately to respiratory and cardiac arrest. Individuals at risk for hypermagnesemia include the elderly, who have decreased renal function and tend to take laxatives, many of which contain magnesium. Additionally, a pregnant patient being treated for eclampsia/toxemia of pregnancy or preterm labor with magnesium is at risk for overdose and toxicity. ⬤

Hypermagnesemia can result from

- Excessive intake of magnesium-containing medications, particularly in the presence of renal insufficiency or failure.

- Excessive infusion of magnesium in the treatment of toxemia of pregnancy or premature labor.

CAUSES AND SYMPTOMS

The most frequent cause of hypermagnesemia is renal failure, particularly with the intake of medications containing magnesium. Elderly patients are at particular risk for magnesium excess owing to decreased renal function and a tendency for increased laxative and antacid use in this population. ⬤ Medications with high levels of magnesium include

- Hydromagnesium aluminate (Riopan, Magaldrate)—antacid
- Magnesium hydroxide (milk of magnesia) and magnesium oxide—laxative
- Magnesium hydroxide and aluminum hydroxide (Maalox)—antacid
- Magnesium salicylate (Doan's pills)—nonnarcotic analgesic
- Magnesium citrate (Citroma, Citro-Nesia)—laxative
- Magnesium sulfate (Epsom salt)—laxative
- Maalox—antacid
- Magnesium sulfate—administered for toxemia of pregnancy/ecampsia

Magnesium excess affects the central nervous system (CNS) and neuromuscular and cardiac systems. People who have hypermagnesemia usually have diarrhea, may feel flushed and drowsy, and perspire profusely. Vomiting, weakness, diminished reflexes, and shallow breathing are other symptoms. The patient's blood pressure drops, and heatbeat slows down considerably. In severe cases, hallucinations, coma, and cardiac arrest can follow. **3**

Magnesium, in elevated levels, has a sedative impact, particularly on nerves and muscles. For example, magnesium may be given in preterm labor to depress uterine contractions or in **eclampsia/toxemia of pregnancy** (a syndrome including proteinuria, edema, and pregnancy-induced hypertension progressing to convulsions) to decrease CNS activity and prevent or minimize convulsions. Symptoms occur most frequently at magnesium levels above 4 mEq/L **4 5** and include

- Flushing
- Nausea
- Vomiting
- Slurred speech
- Lethargy
- Coma
- Cardiac dysrhythmias—bradycardia
- Hypotension
- Respiratory failure
- Death **3 4**

NURSING IMPLICATIONS IN THE TREATMENT OF HYPERMAGNESEMIA

Prevention is the most important nursing responsibility in magnesium management. Patient education, particularly for patients with renal function impairment, should center on limiting the intake of magnesium in foods and medications. Patients and caregivers should be instructed to read the labels of all over-the-counter medications for magnesium content. Also instruct patients to inform any new primary-care provider and notify the pharmacist that the patient has diagnosed renal impairment so that prescription medications with high magnesium levels can be avoided.

Administration of magnesium for CNS depression in cases of premature labor or eclampsia has nursing implications related to watching for signs of hypermagnesemia. Of particular concern is the possibility of respiratory depression secondary to magnesium toxicity. Vital signs, including respiratory rate, depth, and regularity, should be monitored closely during magnesium administration.

If treatment of hypermagnesemia is indicated by the severity of symptoms,

- Intravenous (IV) calcium (i.e., calcium chloride or calcium gluconate) may be administered in an emergency situation to block the action of magnesium.

- Increased fluid intake may be encouraged and provided to promote excretion of magnesium via the kidneys.

- If the patient has impaired renal function, **hemodialysis** (i.e., filtration of the blood through an artificial kidney) may be needed to remove excess magnesium. **6**

SPEED BUMP

1. *Which of the following pieces of clinical information indicates that the patient may be at risk for hypermagnesemia?*

   (a) *Urine output over the last 8 hours was 400 mL/h.*

   (b) *The patient has renal insufficiency and frequent episodes of indigestion.*

   (c) *The patient's sodium level is 120 mEq/L (mmol/L) or less.*

   (d) *The patient reports having nausea and vomiting for the last 4 days.*

2. *Which of the following pieces of information from the patient's history would alert the nurse to watch the patient closely for signs of hypermagnesemia?*

   (a) *The patient was diagnosed with liver inflammation 2 months ago.*

   (b) *The patient is taking furosemide (Lasix) three times a day.*

   (c) *The patient complains of frequent periods of nausea and vomiting.*

   (d) *The patient's occupation involves sitting for long periods.*

3. *The nurse would monitor for which of the following signs that the treatment provided to a patient for hypermagnesemia may be excessive?*

   (a) *The patient is unable to hold a glass of water owing to muscle tremors.*

   (b) *The nurse notes respiratory depression with hypoventilation.*

   (c) *The nurse notes that the patient's urine output is 10 mL/h for 3 hours.*

   (d) *The patient demonstrates weakness, confusion, and lethargy.*

Hypomagnesemia

Decreased serum magnesium levels (i.e., **hypomagnesemia**) occurs when the magnesium concentration in the blood plasma falls below the normal range

(< 1.3 mEq/L or 0.65 mmol/L). Malnutrition is one cause of inadequate magnesium levels, particularly when protein and caloric intake are severely reduced. Alcoholics are at particular risk for hypomagnesemia owing to gastrointestinal malabsorption issues and poor nutritional intake. Low potassium levels may result from hypomagnesemia owing to an increased secretion of potassium when magnesium levels are low. Patients with low blood levels of potassium and calcium will experience significant difficulty with low magnesium levels, and magnesium supplements may be required to reverse these deficits. 🔑 The effects of hypomagnesemia may be increased in the presence of hypokalemia and hypocalcemia because all these states result in neuromuscular irritability.

CAUSES AND SYMPTOMS

Two of the main causes of hypomagnesemia are

- Decreased magnesium absorption in the gastrointestinal (GI) tract
- Excessive excretion of magnesium in the urine (i.e., renal malfunction)

Reduced absorption from the GI tract has many causes, some of which are diarrhea, insufficient dietary intake, damage to the small intestine that may inhibit absorption, and malnutrition. Some common causes of excessive loss in the urine include diureses owing to alcohol, loop diuretics, and glycosuria. Other factors that may lead to hypomagnesemia are hypersecretion of aldosterone (causing hypernatremia), ADH, or thyroid hormone and excessive vitamin D (causing hypercalcemia) and intravenous fluids.

The concentration of magnesium in the blood can fall because of

- A loss of magnesium in the urine (increased in diabetes)
- Protein or calorie malnutrition
- Dehydration
- GI disorders that cause loss or limited absorption of magnesium (e.g., Crohn disease, gluten-sensitive enteropathy, regional enteritis, or fat malabsorption owing to surgery or infection)
- Vomiting and diarrhea
- High alcohol intake or alcoholism (increases loss in magnesium)
- Medications, including
  - Some diuretics (e.g., Lasix, Bumex, Edecrin, and hydrochlorothiazide)
  - Some antibiotics (e.g., gentamicin, amphotericin, and cyclosporine)
  - Some cancer medications (e.g., cisplatin)

Many symptoms of hypomagnesemia are associated with hyperactivity. Symptoms of hypomagnesemia include muscle cramps and weakness, abnormal heart rhythms, and tremors. Some people experience twitching of the eye and abnormal involuntary movements. In cases where the magnesium levels becomes very low, patients may hallucinate, blood pressure and heart rate may increase, and heart rhythm may become abnormal. Severe magnesium deficiency can cause seizures, especially in children. Other symptoms include loss of appetite (with possible weight loss), stool containing a high fat content, restlessness, confusion, and irritability. **5**

The symptoms of hypomagnesemia are primarily neuromuscular and include

- Muscle tremor
- Tetany
- Hyperactive reflexes
- Ventricular irritability
  - Premature ventricular contractions
  - Ventricular fibrillation
- Anorexia
- Nausea and vomiting **3**

NURSING IMPLICATIONS IN THE TREATMENT OF HYPOMAGNESEMIA

The primary treatment for hypomagnesemia is oral supplementation and increased dietary intake of foods containing magnesium. Table 8–1 lists suggested dietary interventions.

If the magnesium level is severely deficient, supplementation is provided intravenously or by intramuscular injection. It is critical that the nurse monitor the magnesium infusion carefully because rapid administration can result in cardiac or respiratory arrest. **6**

Conclusion

Magnesium plays an important role in neuromuscular function, affecting neuromuscular excitability. It is critical to life because it has an impact on cardiac

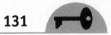

Table 8–1   Suggested Dietary Interventions for Hypomagnesemia

- Dark green vegetables such as spinach (magnesium contained in the center of the chlorophyll molecule)
- Nuts (e.g., cashews and almonds, including peanut butter)
- Seeds
- Chocolate
- Some whole grains (e.g., bran, shredded wheat)
- Variety of foods—five servings of fruits and vegetables (including baked potato with skin and oranges or bananas)
- The magnesium content of refined foods is usually low. Whole-wheat bread, for example, has twice as much magnesium as white bread (magnesium-rich germ and bran are removed when processed).
- Water can provide magnesium, but the amount varies according to the water supply. "Hard" water contains more than "soft" water.
- Recommended daily allowance of magnesium is 400–430 mg for men and 310–360 mg for women, with an extra 40 mg needed for pregnancy.

function as well as respiratory function. Magnesium is also important to the stability of bone. Several key points should be noted from this chapter:

- Magnesium plays an important role in neuromuscular excitability.
- Magnesium is stored primarily in the cells and bone.
- High levels of magnesium result in neuromuscular sedation.
- Low levels of magnesium result in increased neuromuscular excitability.
- Intake of magnesium-containing drugs in the presence of renal insufficiency or failure can result in hypermagnesemia.
- The elderly are at risk for hypermagnesemia.
- Alcoholism and malnutrition can result in decreased magnesium levels.
- Hypernatremia and hypercalcemia can cause a reduction in magnesium absorption.
- Low potassium and low calcium levels can increase the effects of hypomagnesemia.
- Calcium can be administered to counteract the effects of excessive magnesium.
- Overtreatment of one magnesium imbalance could result in the opposite magnesium imbalance

Case Application

A 50-year-old male patient with cirrhosis and a history of alcohol abuse since age 12 is admitted to the emergency room with seizures. He is dehydrated, and the physician has ordered an intravenous infusion of magnesium sulfate to reduce the seizure activity. In addition, the patient has hypertension treated with diuretics. When reviewing the laboratory work, the nurse notices that the serum blood urea nitrogen (BUN) and creatinine are elevated. The nurse also notices that the serum sodium concentration is elevated and the potassium level is low. The patient is in no apparent distress, with vital signs of blood pressure (BP) 110/62 mm Hg, pulse (P) 60 beats/minute, respiration (R) 12 breaths/minute, and pulse oximetry showing 88 percent oxygen saturation.

Considering this case, the nurse should be concerned about what data and monitor for what possible consequences?

- In a patient 50 years old, anticipate that some bodily functions have declined, including renal function.

- Magnesium sulfate likely will accumulate more rapidly than in a younger patient.

- An elevated BUN and creatinine indicate a decrease in renal function, placing the patient at risk for hypermagnesemia.

- Hypernatremia may reduce magnesium reabsorption, but if sodium is lost with diuretics, magnesium reabsorption will not be reduced.

- Although the vital signs are within normal range, the respiratory rate and pulse are both on the lower end of normal and easily could be depressed if magnesium toxicity occurs.

- The vital signs and oxygenation should be monitored continuously.

- A baseline measure of the patella reflex should be obtained by the nurse.

- Reflexes should be monitored often (every 15–30 minutes or as ordered) during the magnesium infusion.

- A loss of deep tendon reflex or any sign of respiratory depression (e.g., decreased depth or rate) or cardiac depression (i.e., bradycardia) should be reported to the primary-care provider immediately.

- Calcium should be kept available for emergency use to block the actions of magnesium.

- Monitor laboratory values and report levels of electrolytes and any imbalances, if noted.

Final Check-up

1. A patient is admitted in delirium tremens. History shows an intake of a quart of alcohol each day. The patient is 30 pounds under weight. The nurse would anticipate which of the following treatments to address the magnesium imbalance the patient is at highest risk for?

   (a) Increased intake of foods such as potato chips to increase sodium level.

   (b) Push 100–150 mL of intravenous fluids hourly to increase diuresis.

   (c) Administer a magnesium supplement by intramuscular injection.

   (d) Administer vitamin D and vitamin B_{12} supplements.

2. The nurse should watch which of the following patients most closely for hypomagnesemia?

   (a) Andy Peters, who eats fresh fruits and vegetables three times each day

   (b) Azara Akbar, who is pregnant and having twins next week

   (c) Lola Ameriz, who has been constipated and is taking laxatives daily

   (d) Bob Green, who is homeless and drinks 1 pint of alcohol each day

3. Bailey McIntosh, age 34, was admitted with dehydration and hypernatremia after a marathon race. The nurse would watch closely for which of the following signs of a likely magnesium imbalance?

   (a) Slow cardiac rate and rhythm

   (b) Respiratory rate below 10 breaths/minute

   (c) Muscle tremors in the extremities

   (d) Blood pressure of 90/58 mm Hg or below

4. The nurse suspects that Mrs. Hong has an elevated magnesium level. Which of the following pieces of information collected in the history would place Mrs. Hong at risk for hypermagnesemia?

   (a) A report of loose stools six to eight times per day for 4 days

   (b) Chronic renal failure and taking Maalox for indigestion

   (c) A past pregnancy resulting in an aldosterone excess

   (d) A recent episode of acute pancreatitis

5. Which of the following symptoms would indicate that the treatment for a patient with hypomagnesemia had been effective?

   (a) The patient's heart rate is 90 beats/minute, and the rhythm is regular.

   (b) The patient's muscle tone and reflexes are hyperreactive.

(c) The patient's lips and mucous membranes are dry.

(d) The patient's urinary output is 30 mL or more per hour.

References

Needham A. *Comparative and Environmental Physiology Acidosis and Alkalosis.* 2004.

Pagana KD, Pagana TJ. *Mosby's Manual of Diagnostic and Laboratory Tests,* 3rd ed. St. Louis: Mosby Elsevier, 2006.

Saladin K. *Anatomy and Physiology: The Unity of Form and Function,* 4th ed. New York: McGraw-Hill, 2007.

Web Site

http://en.wikipedia.org/wiki/Acidosis

CHAPTER 9

Phosphorus Imbalances: Hypophosphatemia and Hyperphosphatemia

Learning Objectives

At the end of this chapter, the student will be able to

1 Describe the process of normal phosphorous metabolism in the human body.

2 State the normal value ranges for serum phosphate levels.

3 Compare and contrast causes, manifestations, and treatments for hypophosphatemia and hyperphosphatemia.

4. Describe diagnostic tests and procedures that are used in making a definitive diagnosis of hypophosphatemia and hyperphosphatemia.

5. Identify special populations at risk for the development of hyperphosphatemia.

6. Differentiate between complications that would be associated with acute hyperphosphatemia versus chronic hyperphosphatemia.

7. Discuss nursing interventions related to the treatment of impaired calcium metabolism.

Key Terms

Anorexia nervosa

Ateriosclerosis

Calcitonin

Crohn disease

Hemolytic anemia

Hyperphosphosphatemia

Hyperventilation

Hypophosphatemia

Malnutrition

Metabolism

Respiratory alkalosis

Rhabdomyolysis

Sepsis

Overview

Phosphorous is an important element in essentially all existing forms of life. In human beings, phosphorous is found predominantly in the form of phosphate. Phosphate is the sixth most abundant mineral in the body and is the most abundant intracellular anion in the body. It provides the energy-rich bonds of adenosine triphosphate (ATP) used for multiple processes in the body, including

- Muscle contractions
- Nerve transmission
- Electrolyte transport

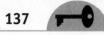

Phosphate plays a key role in

- Energy (i.e., carbohydrate, protein, and fat) **metabolism** (total chemical reactions in the body)
- B-complex vitamins use
- Cell structure
- Genetic coding
- Blood cells
- Acid–base balance

Phosphate is found in all parts of the body but is most abundant in the bones and teeth (85 percent). Phosphate circulates in the blood in a protein-bound form (12 percent), a complexed form (33 percent), and an ionized form (55 percent), which is the physiologically active form. However, most laboratory values represent the total phosphate level. The phosphate level will fluctuate during the day based on physiologic activity that may increase cellular use. The reported level may be low because more phosphate is intracellular than usual or may be high because more phosphate has moved out of the cells than usual in response to some temporary situation. Thus a full assessment is important to ensure that the proper treatment is provided. For example, if phosphate levels are high, calcium levels should be assessed to determine if the elevation might be due to a release of calcium and phosphate from bone. Treatments then are planned to address the actual cause of the imbalance.

1 Phosphorous metabolism is regulated by

- Gastrointestinal (GI) absorption
- Renal excretion
- Cellular regulation
- Hormonal regulation

Most foods contain phosphorous; thus there is usually no problem associated with an inadequate intake. In addition, the GI system is very efficient in the absorption of these mineral, usually absorbing two-thirds of the phosphorous ingested. Additionally, vitamin D increases phosphate absorption in the intestines. Foods that are highest in phosphorus include

- Red meat
- Fish
- Poultry
- Eggs
- Milk products
- Legumes

The usual daily intake of phosphate is between 800 and 1200 mg/day. Absorption of phosphate may be impaired by some medications (e.g., aluminum- and magnesium-based antacids that bind phosphates) or by malabsorption syndrome. Malnourishment may result in low levels of phosphate owing to decreased food intake and decreased vitamin D intake.

The kidneys regulate the excretion of phosphorous and often will excrete up to 90 percent of what is ingested to offset excess accumulation. In the presence of renal insufficiency or failure, high ingestion of phosphate can place the patient at risk for hyperphosphatemia. On the contrary, use of diuretics or renal transplantation after renal failure may result in phophaturia (i.e., loss of phosphate in the urine).

Cellular uptake of phosphate varies with circumstances in the body:

- Hyperglycemia—insulin will increase cellular uptake of phosphate as glucose is driven into the cell.

- Alkalosis—cellular uptake is increased.

- Rewarming after hypothermia—increases cellular uptake of phosphate.

- Stress—increased catecholamine release increases cellular uptake of phosphate.

Cellular depletion of phosphate may be masked by serum levels that are within normal limits, but phosphate return to cells (e.g., during insulin use with hyperglycemia) will reveal the deficit and result in a low serum phosphate concentration.

Hormones from both the parathyroid gland (i.e., parathyroid hormone) and the thyroid gland (i.e., **calcitonin**) regulate the phosphate levels in body fluid. There is often an inverse relationship between phosphate and calcium, where an elevation in phosphate is associated with a decreased calcium level, and vice versa. This is likely related to phosphate-binding properties of calcium, which moves to bone, leaving less free calcium in the serum. While each of these regulators has been described independently, actual regulation depends on the processes working in unison.

- Parathyroid hormone (PTH)—promotes phosphate excretion and inhibits calcium excretion while stimulating calcium absorption in the intestines.

- Calcitonin—antagonizes (blocks) the action of PTH, thus reducing phosphate excretion.

Thus calcium and phosphate levels can affect each other. Other electrolytes, such as magnesium and potassium, also can affect phosphate levels (e.g., hypomagnesium can stimulate phosphate loss in the urine, and hypokalemia, perhaps owing to its association with alkalosis, can stimulate phosphate use by the cells).

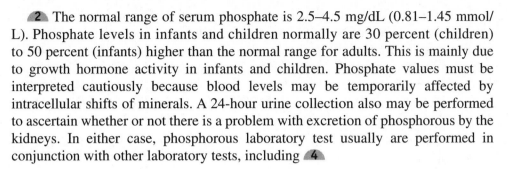 The normal range of serum phosphate is 2.5–4.5 mg/dL (0.81–1.45 mmol/L). Phosphate levels in infants and children normally are 30 percent (children) to 50 percent (infants) higher than the normal range for adults. This is mainly due to growth hormone activity in infants and children. Phosphate values must be interpreted cautiously because blood levels may be temporarily affected by intracellular shifts of minerals. A 24-hour urine collection also may be performed to ascertain whether or not there is a problem with excretion of phosphorous by the kidneys. In either case, phosphorous laboratory test usually are performed in conjunction with other laboratory tests, including

- Calcium
- Electrolyte panel
  - Sodium
  - Potassium
  - Chloride
- Parathyroid hormone
- Vitamin D
- Magnesium

These tests provide a more accurate determination of the significance of the results. A full picture of other imbalances could indicate possible intracellular phosphate deficits.

Hypophosphatemia

CAUSES AND SYMPTOMS

Hypophosphatemia, that is, a low level of phosphorous in the blood, occurs when phosphate levels are below 2.5 mg/dL. The cause is rarely related dietary intake mainly because most foods in the American diet provide more than enough phosphorous.

More often hypophosphatemia occurs secondary to other diseases or conditions.

- Conditions accompanied by **hyperventilation** (above normal respiratory rate and depth), such as diabetic ketoacidosis, **sepsis** (systemic infection), and alcohol withdrawal, result in a shift of phosphate out of the bloodstream into the cells, which, in turn, will cause hypophosphatemia.

- Refeeding syndrome also causes a similar shift of phosphate into the cells. In most cases, refeeding syndrome occurs in patients who are being treated for severe **malnutrition** or starvation. Treatment of such patients involves oral intake of carbohydrates and/or administration of intravenous (IV) fluid. Glucose (i.e., carbohydrates broken down) triggers the release of insulin, which allows entry of glucose into cells but also increases the movement of phosphate into the cells, the outcome again being hypophosphatemia.

- Malabsorption disorders such as **Crohn disease** can decrease absorption of phosphates.

- Ingestion of large amounts of phosphate-binding antacids (aluminum is in most antacids) also can cause hypophosphatemia.

- Vitamin D deficiency is also implicated.

- So is hyperparathyroidism (with release of PTH).

- Use of loop diuretics also has been associated with hypophosphatemia.

3 Any condition that alters the reabsorption of phosphorous by the kidneys also may lead to hypophosphatemia.

5 An individual experiencing mild deficiencies of phosphate will be asymptomatic in most cases. Hospitalized patients are more likely to manifest symptoms, and the presence of symptoms is even more frequent in patients admitted to the intensive-care unit. The most common presenting symptoms are

- Muscle weakness (decreased ATP available)

- Respiratory distress secondary to **respiratory alkalosis** (excess base in the blood due to loss of CO_2 in breathing)

- Hypotension related to cardiac involvement

- Pale skin color as a result of **hemolytic anemia** (low blood cell count due to destraction) of Red blood cells

- Altered mental status ranging from irritability to coma

Most of the symptoms are related to the lack of phosphate for ATP formation for energy. Weakness or inadequate function is noted in the absence of phosphate.

NURSING IMPLICATIONS

The nurse plays a key role in the definitive diagnosis of hypophosphatemia. **3**

- When interviewing a patient, the nurse should include questions that elicit information about the patient's use of alcohol and antacids.

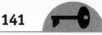

- Teenages are at risk for conditions such as **anorexia nervosa** (eating disorder refusal to take in adequate calories) and should be questioned carefully about dietary habits.

- A list of all medications (i.e., prescription and nonprescription) the patient is currently taken should be obtained to determine if medications that provide excess phosphate or those that stimulate phosphate loss should are being used.

- During the review of systems, the nurse should pay particular attention to the report of conditions such as Crohn disease, diabetes mellitus, and thyroid and kidney disorders owing to the possible impact of these conditions on phosphate absorption and movement into the cell.

- Patients presenting with severe burns are also at greater risk for the development of hypophosphatemia. 5

- Patients being treated for malnutrition should be monitored more closely for hypophosphatemia because of the possible occurrence of refeeding syndrome.

- Particular attention should be paid to serum phosphate levels and the presence of symptoms around the third to fourth days of treatment because hypophosphatemia may not be present initially but may occur within this time frame.

- Motor strength and neurologic and mental status should be assessed. Vital signs also should be monitored closely, with particular emphasis on respiratory rate and pattern and blood pressure.

- Teach the patient about foods containing phosphate. 7

Tips: Keeping Your Phosphorous at the Right Speed

- Get the most phosphorous out of your calories (avoid sodas).
- Prepare foods correctly:
  - Cook for the shortest time possible in a minimal amount of water.
  - Roast or broil lamb, veal, pork, and poultry.
- Eat a variety of foods.
- Consult with your doctor prior to using laxatives and/or enemas.
- Be sensible when exercising.

SPEED BUMP

1. *Which one of the following individuals would be at greatest risk for developing hypophosphatemia?*

    (a) A patient admitted to the intensive-care unit with a diagnosis of respiratory alkalosis

    (b) A teenage patient whose medical history suggests a diagnosis of anorexia nervosa

    (c) A triathlon competitor who engages in strenuous exercise on a regular basis

    (d) A toddler who ingested an overdose of vitamin D

2. *Which of the following responses by the patient, who is to collect a 24-hour urine sample, indicates that he or she understands the correct procedure for collection?*

    (a) Night time urine collection is not necessary.

    (b) The 24-hour time period begins with the first voiding, but the urine for the first voiding should be discarded.

    (c) Urine should be collected at specific intervals depending on the type of test throughout the 24-hour period.

    (d) Water intake should be increased and salt should be restricted during the test.

3. *The normal range for phosphate levels for infants is _____ percent greater than that of adults.*

    (a) 20

    (b) 30

    (c) 40

    (d) 50

Hyperphosphatemia

CAUSES AND SYMPTOMS

Hyperphosphatemia is defined as a blood serum level above 4.5 mg/dL. The most common cause of increased phosphate levels is kidney dysfunction. As mentioned previously, the average American diet has more than enough phosphorous. Consequently, failure of the kidneys to excrete phosphorous at a rate that balances the dietary intake of phosphorous and uptake of phosphorous by the tissues will result in hyperphosphatemia. Other cause of elevated phosphate levels include

- Hypoparathyroidism or pseudoparathyroidism (a condition in which the kidneys lose their ability to respond to PTH)
- Excessive intake of phosphate from food sources, as well as laxatives or enemas that contain phosphate
- Prolonged exercise at a high exertion level, which causes muscle damage and leads to a condition called **rhabdomyolysis**
- Cell destruction from chemotherapy
- Respiratory acidosis
- A deficiency of calcium or magnesium
- Increased vitamin D levels

6 Hypocalcemia occurs secondary to hyperphosphatemia. Most of the signs and symptoms of acute hyperphosphatemia are directly related to the presence of hypocalcemia. Some of these symptoms include

- Numbness
- Tingling
- Muscle spasms
- Tetany
- Seizures (See Chapter 7.)

6 The presence of hyperphosphatemia for extended periods of time may lead to additional manifestations. Calcium deposits in vascular cells may lead to **ateriosclerosis** (hardened arterial walls), which, in turn, will cause increased systolic blood pressure, widening pulse pressure, and eventually hypertrophy of the left ventricle of the heart. When the calcium deposits occur in the peripheral vascular system, the person may develop ulcerations and gangrene in the affected extremities.

---

6 Warning! Dangerous Curve
Renal failure + hyperphosphatemia = calcium deposits

Cardiovascular effects

- Arteriosclerosis
- Hypertension
- Wide pulse pressure
- Left ventricular enlargement
- Cardiac failure
- Increased mortality rate

Peripheral vascular effects

- Ulcerations
- Gangrene

NURSING CONSIDERATIONS

Urgent care of the patient with acute hyperphosphatemia will be geared more toward correction of the coexisting hypocalcemia (refer to "Nursing Implications" for hypocalcemia page 115 in Chapter 7). Most people who have hyperphosphatemia also have end-stage renal disease. Additionally, there is a higher mortality rate among renal disease patients who have chronic hyperphosphatemia. Thus it is very impor-tant that this population of patients be monitored closely for hyperphosphatemia. As with any situation, assessment is foundational to ensuring that the patient has the best outcome. Phosphate and calcium levels should be watched closely. The nurse should report indications of chronic hyperphosphatemia. Renal patients must be strongly encouraged to adhere to the prescribed diet. The patient should be instructed to consult the physician prior to using antacids, laxatives, or enemas. Reassessment of knowledge regarding proper diet and reinforcement of teaching should occur at frequent intervals. Referral to dieticians and support groups geared toward living successfully with renal disease should be requested. The nurse should assist with updating the medical record (e.g., medication changes, laboratory and diagnostic procedure reports, and consult reports) on a regular basis. This is important because these patients have other chronic conditions that may be treated by more than one physician. Maintaining a current and accurate medical record will contribute to the effectiveness of the plan of care and minimize adverse patient outcomes.

Final Check-up

1. Which of the following organs plays a key role in the metabolism of phosphorous?

   (a) Thyroid

   (b) Pituitary

   (c) Hypothalamus

   (d) Adrenal

2. A 27-year-old homeless patient was hospitalized for complications related to starvation. It is now day 4 of his hospitalization. His oral intake of foods has improved, but he remains on intravenous glucose solution. Which of the following findings would suggest that the patient is experiencing a treatment-related complication?

   (a) Phosphorous level > 4.5 mg/dL

   (b) Fruity-smelling breath

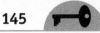

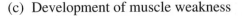

(c) Development of muscle weakness

(d) Bloody stools

3. A patient presents in the emergency department with a tentative diagnosis of chronic hyperphosphatemia. Which of the following clinical findings would be most significant to confirming that the patient has experienced a chronic phosphorous deficit?

    (a) Blood pressure of 170/70 mm Hg

    (b) Pale skin color

    (c) Phosphorous level > 4.5 mg/dL

    (d) Seizure activity

4. Patients with end-stage renal disease who develop hyperphosphatemia have a greater risk of death than those without hyperphosphatemia because of

    (a) increased frequency of seizures.

    (b) respiratory acidosis.

    (c) hemolytic anemia complications.

    (d) cardiovascular complications.

5. Phosphorous plays a key role in which of the following bodily processes?

    (a) Vitamin D absorption

    (b) Vitamin C metabolism

    (c) Energy metabolism

    (d) All the above

6. Which of the following actions by the nurse contributes most significantly to the patient's compliance with the plan of care?

    (a) Maintaining an up-to-date, accurate list of the patient's medications

    (b) Frequent reassessment of the patient's knowledge and reteaching

    (c) Assessment of vital signs at each visit

    (d) Active participation on the treatment team on a regular basis

Web Sites

http://en.wikipedia.org/wiki/Phosphorus
http://labtestsonline.org/understanding/analytes/phosphorus/test.html
www.nlm.nih.gov/medlineplus/ency/article/000307.htm

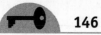

www.nlm.nih.gov/medlineplus/druginfo/natural/patient-phosphorus.html
www.emedicine.com/emerg/topic266.htm
www.emedicine.com/emerg/topic278.htm
www.emedicine.com/med/topic1135.htm
www.hoptechno.com/book29o.htm
www.cc.nih.gov/ccc/patient_education/procdiag/24hr.pdf

CHAPTER 10

Acid–Base Imbalances

Learning Objectives

At the end of this chapter, the student will be able to

1. Compare and contrast acidosis with alkalosis.

2. Identify the source of acidosis or alkalosis based on selected data.

3. Distinguish symptoms of mild and extreme acidosis.

4. Distinguish symptoms of mild and extreme alkalosis.

5. Discuss the potential complications associated with selected acid–base imbalances.

6. Determine the most common electrolyte imbalances associated with prolonged acidosis or alkalosis.

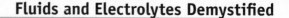

> **Key Terms**
>
> Hypoxemia   pH
>
> Metabolic acidosis   Respiratory acidosis
>
> Metabolic alkalosis   Respiratory alkalosis

Overview

Acid–base balance is critical to homeostasis. The **pH,** a measure of the acidity and alkalinity of a solution, in the body can determine if a required or desired reaction will occur and the effectiveness of that reaction. The enzymes that control the reactions that occur in the body operate under very specific environmental conditions involving temperature and narrow ranges of pH. Metabolism affects and is affected by the pH of body fluids. While the average range of pH in arterial blood lies between 7.35 and 7.45, the blood pH that is compatible with life in mammals is limited to a range between 6.8 and 7.8. If the pH of arterial blood is outside this range, irreversible cell damage can occur.

As stated in the introductory chapters, acid–base balance is focused on regulating the hydrogen ion concentration. **1** When body fluids have an excessive hydrogen ion concentration, the patient is deemed to be in a state of *acidosis*. When the hydrogen ion concentration is low, the patient is in a state of *alkalosis*. Compensation of an acid–base imbalance can occur when the body has partially adjusted, returning the acid–base balance to normal, even though bicarbonate and carbon dioxide levels remain abnormal. The underlying problem must be corrected to fully reverse the imbalance.

Acidosis

When excessive acids (i.e., hydrogen ions) are present in body fluids relative to the bases (i.e., hydroxide ions) or reduced bases/alkali occur relative to the hydrogen ions, the patient is in a state of acidosis. The most common acid in the body is carbonic acid (H_2CO_3). When the patient is in a state of acidosis, the body seeks to buffer or normalize the state by supplying bicarbonate to balance the hydrogen ions. Since the normal ratio of bicarbonate to carbonic acid (i.e., hydrogen ions) is 20:1, any increased acid content changes the ratio, resulting in an acidotic state.

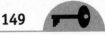

TYPES AND CAUSES OF ACIDOSIS

2 The lungs and kidneys regulate the acid–base status of the body, and increased carbon dioxide, increased body acids, or decreased bicarbonate levels result in acidosis. The causes of acidosis can be categorized as either respiratory, owing to increased CO_2 levels, or metabolic, owing to decreased base or increased production of acids.

Respiratory Acidosis

Respiratory acidosis results when the level of CO_2 in the blood is increased owing to hypoventilation. Slow or shallow breathing decreases the exchange of CO_2 in the lungs and removal of this waste product from the blood. As a prime component of carbonic acid, increased CO_2 causes a shift to the left with higher acid formation and less dissociation of the acid into component parts.

$$H_2O + CO_2 \rightarrow H_2CO_3 \rightleftarrows H^+ + HCO_3^-$$

The determination of respiratory acidosis is made when on blood-gas analysis the pH is lower than 7.35 and the P_{CO_2} is above 45 mm Hg. The CO_2 may be increased in an attempt to balance an alkalotic situation, but the pH, which governs overall state, will indicate the overall state of alkalosis or a normal range if fully compensated.

Causes

2 Pulmonary conditions that result in impaired ventilation will cause a buildup of CO_2. Pulmonary problems, such as chronic obstructive pulmonary disease (COPD), including emphysema, bronchitis, and asthma, and aspiration and severe pneumonia impair the body's ability to remove CO_2. Conditions that suppress respirations, such as head injuries, drugs (especially anesthetics and sedatives), and brain tumors also will decrease CO_2 expiration, resulting in respiratory acidosis.

Metabolic Acidosis

Metabolic acidosis results when there is an excess of acid relative to the base (i.e., bicarbonate) in the body. Additionally, conditions that result in a decreased total amount of base, commonly bicarbonate, relative to the acid in the body will cause metabolic acidosis. Conditions that reduce the ability of the kidneys to excrete acid cause the kidneys to excrete excessive bicarbonate, as well as conditions that result in increased production of acids, will contribute to the development of metabolic acidosis.

Causes

2 Conditions that result in increased production of metabolic acids include lactic acidosis and diabetic ketoacidosis. Lactic acidosis occurs with anaerobic metabolism in the presence of severe **hypoxemia** (i.e., Pao_2 < 36 mm Hg). Any condition that prevents adequate oxygenation resulting in hypoxemia, such as respiratory failure or lung cancer, as well as any condition causing a decrease in perfusion to body tissues, such as heart failure or shock of any form, will result in anaerobic metabolism and lactic acid buildup. In diabetic ketoacidosis, the lack of insulin to move glucose into the cells results in a form of starvation and the production and accumulation of ketoacids (i.e., ketosis) owing to the use of lipids for fuel.

The primary conditions that result in decreased renal excretion of acids and a buildup of metabolic acids are renal disease and renal failure. Additionally, renal disease can result in excessive excretion of bicarbonate. The loss of bicarbonate through diarrhea or overuse of laxative, decreased production of bicarbonate, or ingestion of excessive acid such as acidic poisons, iron, or aspirin could cause metabolic acidosis.

NURSING IMPLICATIONS IN TREATMENT

3 The treatment of respiratory acidosis involves increased ventilation to reduce the CO_2 in the blood. The targets for pH and CO_2 level in patients with chronic lung disease likely will be higher than the normal range. The nurse should monitor for patient's response to treatment, particularly noting laboratory values and vital signs. With ventilation therapy, the nurse should note if the patient's oxygen levels are significantly elevated and if the patient's spontaneous respiratory rate is less than 12 breaths/minute. In some patients with diagnosed or undiagnosed chronic lung disease, respiratory drive may be linked to low oxygen levels; thus elevated oxygen levels that may result from hyperventilation to reduce CO_2 could depress the respiratory drive. Consult with the physician if this is noted.

Treatment of metabolic acidosis is focused on correcting the underlying problem. For example, in lactic acidosis, the correction will center on oxygenation to prevent anaerobic metabolism or fixing other causes of the condition. Similarly, in diabetic ketoacidosis, treatment focuses on correcting the insulin deficit to decrease the burning of fats and production of ketones.

In cases of acidosis in which correction of the underlying respiratory or metabolic cause will be delayed or prolonged, treatment with infusions of bases such as sodium bicarbonate may be used temporarily. Care should be taken not to overtreat the pH, particularly in respiratory acidosis, because the body's actions to correct the problem in combination with infusion of base can result in a metabolic alkalosis and related complications.

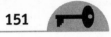

SPEED BUMP

1. *The nurse suspects that Mrs. Agazi has a respiratory acidosis. Which of the following pieces of information would support that suspicion?*

    (a) A decreased pH and a decreased bicarbonate level

    (b) An increased pH and a decreased bicarbonate level

    (c) A respiratory rate below 10 breaths/minute and a pH below 7.30

    (d) An elevated heart rate and a temperature below 96°F

2. *Which client will be at risk for developing acidosis?*

    (a) A woman admitted with constipation

    (b) A child admitted with bowel obstruction

    (c) An infant with Aspirin poisoning

    (d) A man with anxiety and hypertension

Alkalosis

When there is an insufficient concentration of acid (i.e., hydrogen ions) to bind with the bases/alkali (i.e., hydroxide ions) present in body fluids or excessive bases/alkali is present relative to the hydrogen ions, the patient is in a state of alkalosis. The most common base in the body is bicarbonate (HCO_3). When the patient is in a state of alkalosis, the body seeks to buffer or normalize the state by supplying hydrogen ions to balance the bases. Since the normal ratio of bicarbonate to carbonic acid (i.e., hydrogen ions) is 20:1, the absence of sufficient hydrogen ions results in a shift in that ratio to greater concentration of bicarbonate.

TYPES AND CAUSES OF ALKALOSIS

2 Since the lungs and kidneys regulate the acid–base status of the body, decreased CO_2 or increased bicarbonate levels result in alkalosis. The causes of alkalosis can be categorized as either respiratory, owing to decreased CO_2 levels, or metabolic, owing to increased base or decreased acids in the body.

Respiratory Alkalosis

Respiratory alkalosis results when CO_2 levels are decreased owing to increased ventilation. A fast respiratory rate or deep breathing results in the loss of CO_2 from

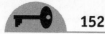

the body. Since CO_2 is the major component of carbonic acid (H_2CO_3), the loss of CO_2 reduces the amount of acid in the body by keeping the reaction moving to the right, leaving more bicarbonate and elevating the pH.

$$H_2O + CO_2 \rightarrow H_2CO_3 \rightleftarrows H^+ + HCO_3^-$$

Causes

Any situation that causes an increase in respiration can result in respiratory alkalosis if the situation persists long enough. Anxiety, if extreme, can cause hyperventilation and loss of CO_2. Low oxygen levels in the blood (i.e., hypoxemia), such as is caused by lung disease or high altitudes (which have lower oxygen levels in the air), can stimulate a patient to breathe faster.

The determination of respiratory alkalosis is made when the pH is above 7.45, and the P_{CO_2} is below 35 mm Hg. The CO_2 may be decreased in an attempt to balance an acidotic situation, but the pH governs the overall state, and thus the CO_2 is being blown off to compensate for an acidotic state. The overall pH may be within normal limits, or if not fully compensated, it may be below 7.35.

Metabolic Alkalosis

Metabolic alkalosis occurs when there is an excess of bicarbonate in the blood owing to increased intake, retention of bicarbonate, or loss of metabolic acids. Bicarbonate is regulated by the kidneys, and any situations that decreases renal excretion of bicarbonate will result in an alkalotic state.

Causes

4 Conditions that stimulate the kidneys to retain bicarbonate will result in alkalosis; for example, in hypochloremia, an extreme lack of chloride, possibly owing to prolonged vomiting, will cause the kidneys to compensate for the chloride loss by conserving bicarbonate. Similarly, extreme hypokalemia, possibly related to diuretic use, will cause the kidneys to react to the lack or loss of potassium by retaining bicarbonate. Hyperaldosteronism can result in increased reabsorption of bicarbonate along with sodium. A loss of gastric acids through vomiting or nasogastric drainage will result in a base excess and alkalosis. Additionally, an excess ingestion of bicarbonate, such as in acid indigestion, will result in alkalosis.

The determination of metabolic alkalosis is made when the pH is above 7.45, and the HCO_3 is above 28 percent. Note that the HCO_3 may be elevated in an attempt to balance an acidotic situation, but the pH governs the overall state. Thus

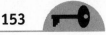

the bicarbonate is being retained to compensate for an acidotic state, and the overall pH may be within normal limits or, if not fully compensated, may be below 7.35.

TREATMENT

Treatment of alkalosis depends on finding the specific cause. For alkalosis caused by hyperventilation, breathing into a paper bag causes more CO_2 to be retained. Oxygen may be administered via a rebreathing mask to prevent decreased oxygenation and hypoxemia. Electrolyte supplements or medications to bind excessive electrolytes may be administered to establish an acid–base balance until the underlying problem has been corrected. Monitor treatment closely and patient responses to avoid overcompensation. Monitor vital signs and laboratory tests because acid–base imbalance and related electrolyte imbalances can result in cardiac dysfunction.

Impact of Acid–Base Imbalances/ Complications

5 Metabolic acidosis can result in stimulation of chemoreceptors, leading to increased ventilatory rate and depth and Kussmaul breathing in an attempt to decrease CO_2 to compensate for the excess acid in the body. If the hyperventilation is prolonged, fatigue could result, leading to respiratory failure.

5 As stated earlier, metabolic alkalosis could result in hypoventilation to reserve CO_2. Prolonged hypoventilation could result in decreased oxygenation and hypoxemia, which would increase acidosis through anaerobic metabolism and lactate production. **6** Additionally, acidosis results in hyperkalemia as H^+ moves into the cell and K^+ moves out of the cell, hypochloremia as Cl^- is lost as ammonium chloride as a buffer for H^+ ions, and hypocalcemia as more calcium binds with protein, leaving less free calcium. Electrolyte imbalances such as those mentioned above result in complications such as neurologic disturbances ranging from irritability to seizures and coma and muscular disturbances, including cardiac dysrhythmia.

Conclusion

Acid–base imbalance has extensive implications for a patient. Treatment of one imbalance could result in another imbalance if care is not exercised. The key to distinguishing between respiratory and metabolic acidosis or alkalosis is that in respiratory acidosis or alkalosis, the CO_2 is increased or decreased, whereas the bicarbonate is either normal (uncompensated) or increased or decreased to balance the pH (compensated). In respiratory or metabolic acidosis or alkalosis, the bicarbonate is high or low, whereas the CO_2 is normal or increased or decreased as compensation for the pH.

Several key points should be noted from this chapter:

- Acid–base balance is important to the metabolic function of the body and optimal function of enzymes.

- There are four types of imbalances, respiratory or metabolic acidosis and respiratory or metabolic alkalosis.

- The pH determines the overall state of acidosis or alkalosis, and assessments of the P_{CO_2} and bicarbonate determine if the source is respiratory or metabolic.

- Overtreatment of an acidosis or alkalosis can result in the opposite imbalance—alkalosis or acidosis.

- Inadequate respiratory function can result in altered acid–base balance and multiple electrolyte imbalances owing to hypoxemia.

- Acid–base imbalances can lead to electrolyte imbalances that can be fatal, specifically imbalances leading to nerve and cardiac dysfunction.

Final Check-up

1. A 50-year-old patient is admitted to the emergency room with chest pain. He states that he is "really scared," and his respiratory rate is 55 breaths/minute, and the breaths are deep. The nurse is unable to calm him and is concerned that he might develop an acid–base imbalance. Which of the following findings would the nurse be likely to observe if the concerns proved to be valid?

    (a) A blood pH of 7.30

    (b) Patient complaints of numbness

    (c) Elevated calcium levels

    (d) Skin that is warm to the touch

2. To determine if a patient has metabolic acidosis, the nurse should assess for which of the following signs or symptoms?

   (a) The cause of or risk factor for hyperventilation

   (b) A pH of 7.49 and an HCO_3 of 22 mEq/L

   (c) A low potassium concentration with dysrhythmia

   (d) A history of prolonged diarrhea

3. Which of the following symptoms indicates a complication that is likely to occur with prolonged acidosis?

   (a) Cardiac dysrhythmia owing to hypokalemia

   (b) Respiratory failure owing to workload on the lungs

   (c) Fluid overload owing to chloride reabsorption and intoxication

   (d) Renal calculi owing to hypercalcemia from protein release of Ca^+

References

Needham A. *Comparative and Environmental Physiology Acidosis and Alkalosis.* 2004.

Pagana KD, Pagana TJ. *Mosby's Manual of Diagnostic and Laboratory Tests,* 3rd ed. St. Louis: Mosby Elsevier, 2006.

Saladin K. *Anatomy and Physiology: The Unity of Form and Function,* 4th ed. New York: McGraw-Hill, 2007.

Web Site

http://en.wikipedia.org/wiki/Acidosis

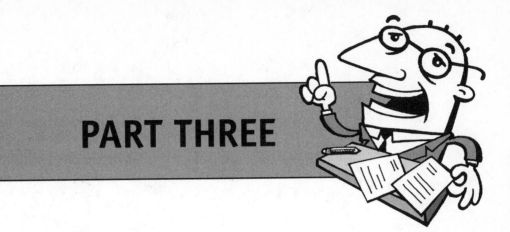

PART THREE

Applications for Fluid and Electrolyte Concepts

CHAPTER 11

Multisystem Conditions Related to Fluid, Electrolyte, and Acid–Base Imbalances

Learning Objectives

At the end of this chapter, the student will be able to

1. Identify aspects of a condition that places the patient at risk for fluid, electrolyte, or acid–base imbalance.

2. Relate the physiologic conditions associated with extreme youth and extreme age that put a patient at high risk for fluid, electrolyte, or acid–base imbalance.

3 Evaluate select conditions for risk factors related to fluid imbalance.

4 Evaluate select conditions for risk factors related to electrolyte imbalance.

5 Evaluate select conditions for risk factors related to acid–base imbalance.

6 Relate symptoms to the identified imbalance(s).

7 Identify diagnostic values associated with imbalances caused by selected conditions.

8 Discuss the potential complications related to treatment of selected conditions.

9 Determine the nursing implications relative to fluid, electrolyte, and acid–base imbalances related to treatment of selected conditions.

Key Terms

Afterload	Hypokalemia
Age extremes	Hyperkalemia
Aldosterone	Hypoproteinemia
Atelectasis	Osteopenia
Burn injury	Osteoporosis
Cardiomyopathy	Pregnancy
Debridement	Preload
Depolarization	Renal insufficiency
Dialysis	Renal failure
Dysrhythmia	Respiratory distress syndrome (RDS)
Hemolysis	Senescence
Hyaline membrane disease	

Overview

Most conditions will cause an imbalance in more than just electrolytes. Fluid imbalance will follow certain electrolyte imbalances, and acid–base imbalance will result from certain electrolyte imbalances. As stated in previous chapters, acid–base imbalances can cause and result from electrolyte imbalances. With this in mind, the nurse must think about all levels of imbalance and anticipate problems that might occur. This is particularly important when treatments for one condition place the patient at risk for another condition or treatment for one imbalance places the patient at risk for the opposite electrolyte, fluid, or acid–base imbalance. Since conditions are multifactorial and involve multiple systems, the nurse must think in terms of multisystem reality and consider that multiple imbalances can and often do occur simultaneously in one patient.

Symptoms and history can be invaluable when determining what imbalances may be present in a patient. The nurse must ask questions to obtain details of dietary practices, exercise habits, work environment, and personal habits such as smoking or drinking to determine if the patient is at risk for conditions that have, up to this point, been undiagnosed. Providing this historical data, along with admission laboratory results and physical assessment data, can assist the primary-care provider in making a diagnosis and will help the nurse advocate for the patient to minimize complications that could worsen the patient's condition. Symptoms can be confusing because many symptoms are shared by several electrolyte or acid–base imbalances and can be present *owing to* a combination of imbalances. Gathering as much historical information as possible could help to distinguish the imbalances that are most likely present and guide the laboratory testing and treatment ordered.

Understanding the normal ranges of electrolytes, arterial blood gases, and other laboratory test values is critical to determining what is important and essential data to report and act on. Laboratory data often will be included as a routine part of the patient's treatment to monitor effectiveness. Close monitoring of laboratory values by the nurse in concert with the medication or treatment administration can prevent overcompensation for one imbalance that might cause another imbalance. Whenever possible, the nurse should be aware of laboratory results *before* administering the medication or fluid challenge. If the nurse has standing orders or the authority to order or perform screening diagnostic tests, such as a urine osmolality or sending a blood sample for electrolyte determination, particularly potassium, he or she should obtain the urine or blood for these tests and note the results in advance of administering treatment. In many cases, an ounce of prevention can be worth a pound of treatment or cure.

This sampling of conditions will not address all conditions the nurse must be alert for as placing the patient at risk for fluid, electrolyte, and acid–base imbalances. These are examples of some common conditions known to cause imbalances. The reader should review these conditions and consider how other conditions may affect similar organs of the body or similar functions in the body and place the patient at risk for fluid, electrolyte, or acid–base imbalances. **1**

Age Extremes

While an age extreme does not qualify as a disease or illness state, certain physiologic differences that accompany extreme youth or extreme age can place a patient at risk for fluid, electrolyte, and acid–base imbalances. The nurse should be aware of risk factors for young (newborn) or elderly (> 65 years of age) patients and take steps to avoid imbalances when possible or work with the primary-care provider to promote early treatment of imbalances when needed. The changes discussed here are not guaranteed to occur in every young or elderly patient but are possible risk factors that may predispose the patient to imbalances.

NEWBORNS

Newborns have less developed function of some organs at birth, with premature infants being at greatest risk for demonstrating diminished organ function. The most common organ function that is not fully developed is that of the kidneys. Additionally, the respiratory function of premature infants may be diminished, as well as the function of the liver. The complications associated with diminished organ function can result in a number of fluid, electrolyte, and acid–base imbalances. The nurse should be alert for these imbalances. **1**

Renal System

- The kidneys are not fully developed at birth and have a decreased ability to concentrate the urine.
- Water loss is high, and the need for fluid intake is high for body weight relative to that of an adult.
- The potential for dehydration is increased for an infant owing to fluid loss.
- The potential for hypernatremia is increased owing to dehydration and hemoconcentration. **1**

Thus the nurse should monitor intake and output, weight, and signs of dehydration.

Respiratory System

- Lung function may be diminished in premature infants.
- **Hyaline membrane disease,** also referred to as **respiratory distress syndrome (RDS),** is a deficiency of pulmonary surfactant resulting in

alveoli collapse (i.e., **atelectasis**) with exhalation and requires great effort for reinflation.

- Should the atelectasis be unresolved, the patient is at risk for decreased gas exchange, which could result in a risk for hypoxia and anaerobic metabolism with lactic acidosis.

- Decreased gas exchange also could result in carbon dioxide buildup with a resulting respiratory acidosis. **1**

Liver

- Diminished liver function might be demonstrated in a premature infant. The primary deficit resulting from decreased liver function is the inability to synthesize adequate amounts of the protein albumin.

- The lack of intravascular albumin results in low protein in the blood (i.e., **hypoproteinemia**) and would decrease the osmotic pressure that draws fluid into the blood vessels. As a result, fluid remains in the tissues and causes edema.

- If a significant amount of fluid is lost into the tissues, hypovolemia could result.

- An additional concern related to immature liver function is the decreased ability to process medications; thus medication may affect the patient to a greater degree than adult patients. Side effects of medications are more prevalent, along with the accompanying fluid, electrolyte, and acid–base imbalances. **1**

ELDERS

As patients age toward later life, degenerative changes that occur in an organ system after the age of peak efficiency (i.e., **senescence**) is noted. Senescence includes

- A gradual loss of reserve capacity
- Reduced healing ability
- A decreased compensation for stress
- Increased susceptibility to disease

Organ systems degenerate at different rates, with some (e.g., the nervous system) reducing in function only by 10 to 15 percent from ages 30 to 80 and others (e.g., the kidneys) reducing as much as 60 percent in function. The specific changes noted in senescence that affect fluid, electrolyte, and acid–base balance are as follows.

Integumentary System

- Skin loses elasticity owing to atrophy of sebaceous glands and loss of collagen. The loss of elasticity makes assessment of skin turgor difficult for dehydration determination.

- Cutaneous vitamin D production is diminished as much as 75 percent, contributing to calcium deficiency with related muscle weakness and slowed neurotransmission.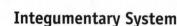

Skeletal System

- **Osteopenia** (i.e., loss of bone) and **osteoporosis** (i.e., porous, fragile bone) are noted owing to osteoclasts (i.e., bone-resorbing cells) that are more active than osteoblasts (i.e., bone depositing cells), resulting in decreased bone density and increased bone fragility

- The impact of calcium deficit (i.e., hypocalcemia) on bone may be greater owing to the preexisting bone loss.

Muscular System

- Replacement of lean body mass with fat and loss of adenosine triphosphate (ATP), creatine phosphate, glycogen, and myoglobin leave muscles weaker.

- The impact of potassium, sodium, or calcium imbalance must be assessed carefully based on the patient's baseline muscle strength and neuromuscular efficiency.

- Historical data are key to establish a patient's ability compensate for prior to electrolyte imbalances and to determine realistic goals and outcomes of treatment.

Nervous System

- Peak efficiency of the nervous system is noted around age 30.

- After age 75, the brain weighs 56 percent less and has fewer synapses, less efficient synaptic transmission, and less neurotransmitter production.

- The impact of potassium, sodium, or calcium imbalance must be assessed carefully based on the patient's baseline muscle strength and neuromuscular efficiency.

- The impact of electrolyte imbalance on the nervous system may be greater in the elderly than in the young owing to the preexisting diminished neurologic function.

- Sensory organ function diminishes, most notably the sense of taste, which migh affect dietary intake leading to malnutrition and decreased protein intake with related fluid balance issues, as well as electrolyte imbalance, in addition to anemia that could affect oxygenation and acid–base balance (lactic acidosis).
- Diminished response to antidiuretic hormone (ADH) stimulation of thirst results in decreased oral intake of fluids and dehydration. **1**

Cardiovascular System

- The cardiac wall becomes thinner and weaker, with decreased stroke volume and cardiac output, resulting in decreased tissue perfusion, including the kidneys.
- Poor renal perfusion could result in renal damage and fluid, electrolyte, and acid–base imbalances.
- Anemia resulting from decreased production of erythropoietin (renal system) and decreased vitamin B_{12} absorption (gastrointestinal system) can result in decreased oxygenation and tissue hypoxia (lactic acidosis).
- Diminished thirst response results in dehydration and decreased circulatory volume and cardiac output.
- Degenerative changes to veins cause valves to weaken and blood to pool in the lower extremities, decreasing venous return and stroke volume and also causing increased pressure in the veins with decreased return of fluid from the tissues and resulting edema.
- Assessment of fluid balance requires baseline historical data relative to edema present in the extremities prior to any suspected fluid imbalance.
- Arterial wall hardening and build up of plaque on the axterial lining results in increased. **Afterload** (Pressure the heart must pump against to push blood out to body systems).

Respiratory System

- Ventilatory function begins to decline after the 20s, with slow but regular loss of lung elasticity and thoracic joint flexibility and loss of cartilage, pulmonary muscle weakening, and a decreased number of alveoli.
- Vital capacity, respiratory volume, and expiratory volume decrease.
- Cough becomes weaker, decreasing clearance of secretions.

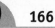

- Chronic obstructive pulmonary disease (COPD) with increased secretions and decreased airway size leads to airway blockage, decreased gas exchange, and hypoxia, which leads to lactic acidosis and carbon dioxide buildup with respiratory acidosis.

- Respiratory effectiveness is decreased, with less capacity to handle a prolonged increase in workload that may be caused by metabolic acidosis.

- Prolonged respiratory compensation for metabolic acidosis is more likely to result in respiratory compromise and eventual failure in an older patient than in a younger patient. **1**

Digestive System

- Decreased taste and decreased saliva (with accompanying difficulty swallowing) contribute to malnutrition, protein deficits, and accompanying fluid imbalance and anemia with circulatory and oxygenation concerns.

- Gastric and intestinal mucosae atrophy with decreased production of acid and intrinsic factor needed for absorption of vitamin B_{12}. These changes result in acid–base imbalance and potential circulatory/respiratory problems related to anemia (i.e., hypoxia). **1**

Renal System

- From the mid-20s to the mid-80s, the number of nephrons (the primary functional cells of the kidney) declines by up to 40 percent.

- The approximately 60 percent remaining cells are less efficient, with decreased blood flow to the cells and decreased glomerular filtration.

- Baseline renal function is maintained, but no reserve capacity is present, leaving the kidneys vulnerable to increased stress or workload owing to increased waste production (or increased electrolytes that must be filtered).

- The kidneys become less sensitive to ADH; thus water is not managed as well, leading to excess loss and dehydration.

- The dehydration is aggravated by the lack of thirst response in the elderly, resulting in decreased intake of fluids and increased serum osmolality and hypernatremia.

- Diminished renal function results in a decreased ability to process medications; thus medication may affect the patient to a greater extent than younger patients. Side effects of medications are more prevalent, along with the accompanying fluid, electrolyte, and acid–base imbalances.

Thus it is evident that patients of extreme youth (newborns) and extreme age (elders) are at greater risk for fluid, electrolyte, and acid–base imbalances. These patients are at greater risk for complication related to these imbalances owing to the preexisting diminished organ function associated with age. **1**

Case Application

An example of the impact of an age extreme on planning for and providing appropriate patient care is found in the situation of Mr. Suarez, age 82, admitted to the hospital on June 15 with altered mental status. In the admission history, the nurse learns that Mr. Suarez lives alone in his own home.

Assessment data: Laboratory values reveal a hematocrit of 40 percent, and Mr. Suarez has a dry tongue and mucous membranes and poor skin turgor when the skin over the forehead is pinched. The sample obtained for admission urinalysis is small in amount (50 mL) and golden in color. The nurse decides to note the electrolyte levels when available, particularly the sodium level.

Interpretation: The nurse suspects dehydration because of the dry tongue and mucous membrane and concentrated urine and remembers that elders are prone to inadequate oral intake owing to a diminished thirst impulse mechanism.

Nursing intervention: Oral fluids are offered (120 mL/h), and within 24 hours, Mr. Suarez is awake and oriented. The sodium level was noted as 144 mEq/L (144 mmol/L) in the admission laboratory tests, and the level was decreased to 138 mEq/L (138 mmol/L) after hydration. The primary-care provider orders an intravenous dextrose solution at 100 mL/h. The nurse monitors intake and output and continues to offer fluids between meals but with lesser frequency (60 mL every 2–3 hours). **9**

Further exploration: Assess the patient's habits to determine possible need for teaching. When asked, Mr. Suarez admits that he seldom drinks more than a cup of coffee (12 oz) for fluids each day, and lately, he has been working in the garden in the heat of the day. **9**

Follow-up assessments and monitoring: The nurse watches Mr. Suarez closely for fluid balance, including urine output (becoming lighter gold in color with hydration, 30 mL/h) and weight (4.4 kg below his normal range on admission but now only 3 kg below the normal range), and continues checking intake and outputs. The nurse also watches for signs of anemia (realizing that the hematocrit was within range because the patient was hemoconcentrated, and after rehydration, the level likely will drop). The nurse also watches for signs of hypervolemia because the patient's fluid therapy could become excessive and overload the patient, particularly because cardiac function diminishes with age, and the patient's heart may have difficulty handling the increased volume. **9**

Evaluation and continued care: The nurse performs full assessments every 12 hours, but notes breath sounds and watches for jugular vein distension (monitoring for rales in the lungs as a sign of left-sided heart overload or jugular venous distension as a sign of right-sided heart overload). As Mr. Suarez's mucous membranes begin to look moist and his urine color becomes clear and pale yellow, the nurse stops pushing fluid between meals and continues to monitor fluid status. Intravenous fluids are decreased to 40 mL/hour. **4**

The nurse must be particularly astute when evaluating symptoms and the impact of treatments. Historical data are key, with appropriate inquiry targeted toward risk factors for the suspected condition. Similarly, a regular and thorough physical examination and monitoring of all systems to promote prevention or early complications are important aspects of care. Since patients are multifaceted, the nurse must monitor all systems to detect areas of concern or areas of potential complications.

SPEED BUMP

1. *Wilson Berry was born 2 months premature. The primary-care provider should be notified of which of the following symptoms indicating that Wilson has inefficient organ function?*

   (a) Pale yellow urine in urine bag

   (b) Arterial blood gases showing a pH of 7.40

   (c) Rales noted in the lungs

   (d) Skin that is pink and returns color in 2 seconds when blanched

2. *Which of the following pieces of information in an 82-year-old patient's history would alert the nurse most to watch the patient closely for signs of hyperkalemia?*

   (a) The patient has reported urinating once every other day.

   (b) The patient is taking furosemide (Lasix) three times a day.

   (c) The dietary history reveals a high intake of fruit and vegetables.

   (d) The occupation history indicates sedentary work inside the home.

Renal Conditions

The renal system plays an important role in the regulation of fluids and electrolytes and is one of the two major systems involved in restoration of acid–base balance. In addition, the renal system has other vital roles, such as production of erythropoetin needed for red blood cells health, essential for oxygenation of tissues. The primary functions of the renal system are

- Filtering the blood to remove excess fluid, electrolytes, and waste products
  - Effectiveness of blood filtration is determined by the glomerular filtration rate (GFR), which is affected by the perfusion to the kidneys and other factors.
  - Filtration is regulated by glomerular blood pressure, which is autoregulated, affected by sympathetic control and hormonal regulation.
    - Autoregulation mechanisms do not fully prevent changes in GFR.
    - The sympathetic nervous system stimulates the release of epinephrine and causes vasoconstriction, reducing perfusion of the kidneys when blood volume is low, reducing the GFR and causing retention of fluid.
    - Hormonal control includes the renin–angiotensin mechanism, which stimulates **aldosterone** (hormone that causes sodium retention) and ADH release to conserve fluid and sodium and stimulates thirst to increase fluid intake.
- Regulating acid–base balance through retention or excretion of bicarbonate
  - In states of acidosis, H^+ ions are excreted, and bicarbonate is retained.
  - In states of alkalosis, H^+ ions are retained, and bicarbonate is excreted.

The renal system is composed of functional units called *nephrons*. Nephrons have two portions, the cortex (i.e., glomerulus, Bowman capsule, and proximal and distal tubules) and the medulla (i.e., the loop of Henle and the collecting tubules). The nephron also contains two primary sections:

- *Renal corpuscle*—contains the glomerular capsule, which is vascular and plays a critical role in filtration of the blood
- *Renal tubules*—the duct leading away from the glomerulus and toward the renal medulla and collecting ducts

Fluids, electrolytes, and bicarbonate are secreted, reabsorbed, and excreted in different areas of the nephron. Additionally, drugs administered to remove or retain fluids or electrolytes are targeted to specific areas of the nephron.

(reabsorption of Na^+, K^+, Ca^{2+}, Mg^{2+}, Cl^-, HCO_3^-, H_2O, some acids and wastes)
(reabsorb H_2O)

Glomerulus → proximal tubule → descending nephron loop

(secretion of H^+, NH_4^+, some drugs, waste and acids)   (secrete urea)

→ ascending nephron loop (Na^+, K^+, Cl^- reabsorption),

→ distal tubule (Na^+, H_2O, Cl^-, HCO_3 reabsorption) and (H^+, K^+, NH_4^+ secretion)

→ collecting tubule (H_2O and urea reabsorption)

If renal function is impaired, the patient is at risk for multiple imbalances. Renal function can be disrupted in different degrees. **Renal insufficiency** is a state in which the kidney, owing to damage and loss of nephrons, cannot sustain homeostasis. Renal insufficiency can be temporary, with recovery of efficient function when the kidney regenerates or other nephrons take over the lost function. If the damage is extensive or ongoing, the insufficiency will progress to total **renal failure.**

Renal failure can be *acute*—rapid loss of renal function owing to kidney damage from such conditions as prolonged hypotension or hypovolemia or owing to nephrotoxic drugs. The key manifestations of acute renal failure (ARF) are

- *Azotemia*—accumulation of nitrogenous waste products such as urea nitrogen and creatinine
- *Uremia*—condition in which symptoms of renal function decline and are noted in multiple systems
- *Oliguria*—urine output below 400 mL/day, although about half the patients will have normal or increased urinary output
- *Fluid and electrolyte imbalance*—hyperkalemia and edema may not be noted initially

The causes of renal failure are varied and can be categorized as being

- *Prerenal*—decreased blood flow to the kidneys, leading to decreased renal tissue perfusion.
- *Intrarenal*—conditions that damage renal tissue, such as nephrotoxic drugs, hemoglobin, myoglobin (as might occur with burn damage), or prolonged ischemia. Causes include acute tubular necrosis (ATN), glomerulonephritis, toxemia of pregnancy, and systemic lupus erythematosus (SLE).

- *Postrenal*—blockage of urinary outflow results in a backup of urine and waste, impairing kidney function. The most common causes are tumors, prostate cancer, trauma, or calculi.

Acute renal failure proceeds in phases, including

- *Initiating phase*—beginning with the assault and proceeding until symptoms occur.
- *Oliguric phase*—usually occurring within 1–7 days and lasting up to 2 weeks. The longer the duration, the more likely the condition will progress to chronic renal failure.
  - Symptoms become evident—urinary changes, fluid volume excess, metabolic acidosis, electrolyte imbalance, waste buildup, and neurologic disorders (Table 11–1).
- *Diuretic phase*—increase in urine output to 1–3 L/day (occasionally up to 3–5 L/day) owing to osmotic diuresis and inability of tubules to concentrate urine.
- *Recovery phase*—GFR increases with clearance of waste and reduction of BUN and creatinine. May take a year to stabilize, with some residual renal insufficiency, and some patients progressing to chronic renal failure.

Chronic renal failure or chronic kidney disease involves progressive and irreversible loss of kidney function. Kidney function progresses from less than half normal to end-stage failure with only one-tenth the normal GFR.

At various stages of renal failure, imbalances in fluids, electrolytes, and acid–base status are noted. In acute renal failure, symptoms may occur suddenly, last for a period of time, and then resolve with treatment (although some residual loss of function may remain). However, in chronic renal failure, imbalances are ongoing and require regular treatment to maintain stability. The manifestations of renal failure are similar, whether acute or chronic, depending on the underlying cause, but chronic renal failure evidences a progressive loss of renal cells that affects several body functions.

The decreased clearance of waste materials results in a buildup of waste in the blood. Blood urea nitrogen (BUN) and creatinine are two end products of protein and muscle metabolism. In addition to waste buildup, electrolyte and acid buildup and bicarbonate loss may be noted, leading to imbalances. Supplemental cleansing of the blood through **dialysis**—use of an artificial kidney (hemodialysis) or the peritoneal membrane (peritoneal dialysis) to filter blood—may be performed until renal function is restored.

The primary manifestations of renal failure and usual treatments are listed in Table 11–1. While treatment of acute renal failure centers on eliminating the underlying cause, managing symptoms, and preventing complications, the care provided in both acute and chronic renal failure is similar for the body systems affected.

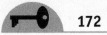

Table 11–1   Primary Manifestations of Acute Renal Failure and Recommended Treatment Regimens

Body System Affected	Manifestation Noted with Renal Failure	Treatment Regimen
Urinary system	• Decreased urine output • Increased urine output (in diuretic phase of acute renal failure—waste clearance remains limited) • Proteinuria • Decreased urine specific gravity (to fixed at 1.010) • Decreased osmolality • Increased urinary sodium	• (Resolve hypovolemia and restore renal perfusion) • Diuretic therapy—loop diuretics, osmotic diuretics • Volume expanders • Early and frequent dialysis • Monitor for hypervolemia in oliguric phase and hypovolemia in diuretic phase • Weight daily (1 kg weight equivalent to 1000 mL fluid)
Respiratory system	• Pulmonary edema • Kussmaul respirations (to decrease CO_2 to balance metabolic acidosis)	• Fluid management to reduce overload • Treatment of metabolic acidosis
Metabolic system	• Increased BUN and creatinine owing to decreased waste clearance • Decreased sodium, calcium, pH, and bicarbonate • Increased potassium and phosphate	• Dialysis therapy—fluid and electrolytes move from higher gradient (blood) to lower gradient in dialysate (fluid infusing around semipermeable membrane or exchange) • Dietary restrictions based on patient's lab work (see GI) • Potassium level reduction—insulin and glucose drive potassium into cell (temporary) • Sodium bicarbonate to treat acidosis owing to K^+ shift • Calcium gluconate to raise the threshold for excitability and decease dysrhythmia • Intake and output • Weight daily (1 kg weight equivalent to 1000 mL fluid)
Cardiovascular system	• Volume overload (renal retention of fluids) • Heart failure—jugular venous distension, edema • Hypotention (early stage) • Hypertension (with fluid overload) • Pericarditis and pericardial effusion • Dysrhythmia (electrolyte imbalances and waste)	• Fluid restrictions (600 mL + fluid loss over previous 24 hours) • Dialysis • Potassium level reduction • Calcium gluconate to raise the threshold for excitability and decease dysrhythmia

(Continued)

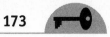

Table 11-1   Primary Manifestations of Acute Renal Failure and Recommended Treatment Regimens
(Continued)

Body System Affected	Manifestation Noted with Renal Failure	Treatment Regimen
Neurologic system	Neurologic changes owing to electrolyte imbalance and waste • Lethargy • Seizures • Asterixis • Memory impairment	• Hemodialysis • Dietary restrictions (see GI) • Calcium supplements or phosphate-binding agent • Potassium level reduction
Gastrointestinal system	• Nausea and vomiting • Diarrhea • Constipation • Anorexia • Stomatitis (waste buildup) • Bleeding (waste buildup, impaired clotting)	• Parenteral nutrition (if indicated) • Enteral nutrition (if indicated) • Dietary restriction of potassium (40 mEq or as ordered), sodium, phosphate based on values of labwork • Protein intake based on need (0.6–2 g/kg/day)

Case Application

Pearl Jones was admitted to the intensive-care unit after a car accident with approximately 3 L of blood loss three days ago. She is semiconscious but irritable and has a blood pressure (BP) of 92/40 mm Hg, pulse (P) of 140 beats/minute, and respiration (R) of 38 breaths/minute, and her skin is cool and pale with pale mucous membranes. Arterial blood-gas analysis reveals a pH of 7.32, Pco_2 of 33 mm Hg, O_2 of 70 percent, and HCO_3 of 14 mEq/L. Urine output is 200 mL for the past 24 hours. Diagnostic tests ordered include an electrolyte panel (Na^+, K^+, Cl^-, and CO_2). What additional data would be beneficial to determine care measures for Ms. Jones?

Suggested areas to explore include

- What were the patient's vital signs over the past 3 days, and for what length of time was the patient without treatment after the accident? *This indicates the total time kidneys may have been exposed to hypovolemia and hypotension.*

- Does the patient have any other conditions? *Heart disease, renal insufficiency, diabetes, or endocrine conditions (e.g., Cushing, hyperaldosteronism, diabetes insipidus, or SIADH), which could place the patient at high risk for fluid overload, dehydration, or electrolyte imbalance when combined with the current assault.*

- What are the values for the electrolytes, and in addition, what are the current values of the patient's calcium, phosphate, BUN, and creatinine? *Imbalances could indicate renal failure and stage of renal failure present.*

- What is the patient's urine specific gravity? *If the value is low or fixed, it indicates loss of renal ability to concentrate urine and clear waste.*

- What does the physical assessment reveal?

  - Breath sounds? *Rales could indicate pulmonary edema, and tachypnea indicates compensation for metabolic acidosis.*

  - Cardiovascular—jugular venous distension, edema, skin cool and pale, with decreased capillary refill (> 4 seconds)? *Signs of hypovolemia and possible heart failure, hypertension may be present if fluid overload is intravascular.* Is heart rhythm regular or irregular? What does the electrocardiogram (ECG) show? *Could indicate electrolyte imbalance.*

  - Gastrointestinal—absent bowel sounds, vomiting, or diarrhea? *Could indicate electrolyte imbalance (e.g., hypocalcemia or hyper/hypokalemia).*

- What treatments might the nurse anticipate and with what complications?

  - Diuretics with albumen infusions to return fluid to intravascular area and remove excessive fluid.

  - Electrolyte monitoring with replacement of calcium and sodium as indicated, removal of potassium, and binding of phosphate, if indicated. *Monitor for excess or deficient electrolyte levels.*

  - Dialysis. *Monitor closely for fluid and electrolyte shifts owing to dialysate. Watch vital signs carefully.*

  - Cardiovascular medications to control hypertension and **dysrhythmia,** (irregular on abnormal cardiac Rhytham or rate) if indicated. *Monitor blood pressure and pulse rate and regularity to determine if heart is excessively depressed.*

If Ms. Jones' urine output increases to 2000 mL per 24 hours, the nurse should perform what exploration to determine the degree of the patient's recovery?

- Measure the specific gravity of urine specimen. *Determine if kidneys are clearing waste materials.*

- Assess laboratory values. *Determine if creatinine level is decreasing.*

- Monitor for hypokalemia, hyponatremia, and signs of dehydration (hematocrit levels). *To determine if fluids and electrolytes are normalizing.*

The role of the nurse in acute or chronic renal failure is focused on anticipating and preventing further renal damage by restoring renal perfusion, detecting and reporting early signs of renal dysfunction, and providing treatments promptly. Since treatment of fluid and electrolyte imbalance can result in the opposite imbalance, close monitoring of patient status is important to restoring and maintaining homeostasis.

SPEED BUMP

1. When the patient is in the oliguric phase of renal failure, what treatment would be appropriate?

   (a) Potassium supplements and increased intake of green vegetables

   (b) A high-phosphate diet with supplements as indicated

   (c) Dialysis therapy with dialysate that is low in potassium

   (d) Diet restricting dairy products to reduce intake of calcium.

2. The nurse would monitor for what signs that the treatment provided to a patient for hyperkalemia may be excessive?

   (a) The patient has absent bowel sounds with nausea and vomiting.

   (b) The patient demonstrates anxiety and irritability.

   (c) The urine output remains 30 mL/h for 3 hours.

   (d) The patient's ECG has peaked T waves and a wide QRS complex.

Conditions with High Impact on Fluid Balance: Burn Injury and Pregnancy

BURN INJURY

The integumentary system (i.e., the skin) serves multiple functions in preserving homeostasis. Several of these functions, if disrupted, could result in fluid volume imbalance. The skin also provides invaluable data related to disturbance in sensory or circulatory status. Any injury to the skin, such as a laceration or tearing from trauma or friction, will disrupt the function of the skin. Five main physical functions of the skin include

- Resistance to trauma and infection by keeping most trauma and friction at the surface and keeping organisms at the surface and away from the bloodstream.

- Other barrier functions, particularly barrier to water to prevent absorption of excess water. In addition, skin protects the body from ultraviolet radiation, as well as from some chemicals, by limiting the exposure to the upper layers of skin, not deeper tissue.

- Vitamin D synthesis. The first step in this process begins at the skin level, and the process is completed in the liver and kidneys. Vitamin D is essential to calcium levels.

- Sensation. The skin holds nerve endings that react to temperature, touch, texture, vibration, pressure, and tissue injury. The skin provides an early warning system to tell the brain to withdraw from noxious/harmful stimuli before serious tissue damage is done.

- Thermoregulation. The skin helps to retain heat when cold is sensed through vasoconstriction and decreased circulation to the skin to reduce exposure of blood to cold and responds to hot temperatures by releasing heat through vasodilation. The skin contains sweat glands that allow heat and moisture (99 percent water) to escape the body to cool the individual.

Burn injury represents the destruction of a portion of the skin owing to intense heat, contact with a caustic chemical, or electricity. Burn injury is classified based on the depth of the injury:

- *First degree*—involving only the epidermis
- *Second degree*—also called *partial-thickness injury,* involving the epidermis and part of the dermis
- *Third degree*—also referred to as *full-thickness injury,* involving the epidermis, dermis, and deeper tissue, including muscle on some occasions

Additional injury that occurs in burns includes smoke and inhalation injury. Numerous consequences are associated with burn injury. The degree of injury and impact of the burn will be higher for children than for adults with the same percentage of body surface area burned (Fig. 11–1). Since children have more fluid content in the body, fluid loss is more critical. In addition, respiratory airways are smaller in children than in adults, and therefore airway blockage is a higher risk.

This section will focus on damage affecting fluid, electrolyte, and acid–base balance.

Fluid

The primary concern in a burn injury patient is the sequence of events resulting in fluid shifts from the vasculature to extravascular spaces. When the skin barrier is damaged, a set of events occurs that includes an inflammatory response involving

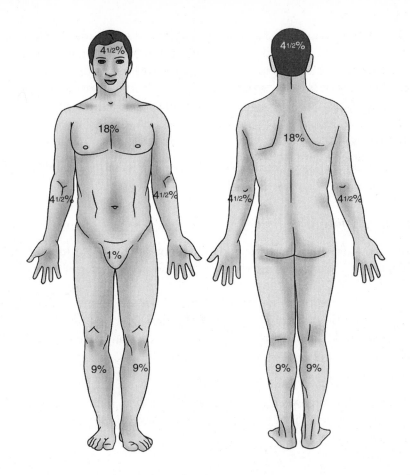

Figure 11–1   "Rule of nines" for an adult. Head and neck, 9 percent; arms (each),
9 percent; anterior trunk, 18 percent; posterior trunk, 18 percent; legs (each), 18 percent;
and perineum, 1 percent. Total, 100 percent.

vasodilation and fluid and nutrients moving to the area to begin the healing process.
Because large areas of the skin are affected, however, the fluids are lost from the
body through the open wounds. **3**

> Burn injury → increased vascular permeability → fluid into tissues (edema) and
> decreased intravascular volume → hemoconcentrated blood and increased viscosity
> (high hematocrit) → loss of protein (albumin) and decreased oncotic pressure in
> veins → further loss of fluid from vessels to interstitial tissues → hypovolemic shock

The degree of fluid loss is related to the extent of skin damage. The inflammatory response may continue for up to 48 hours before the shift in fluids begins to reverse. Large volumes of fluid are lost to the interstitial spaces initially in addition to wound drainage. The nurse is focused on restoration of fluid volume to prevent progression to irreversible shock, as well as monitoring intake and output to prevent further fluid volume deficit or volume overload. In addition, the peripheral circulation is monitored because the viscous blood causes obstructions in the microcirculation. Volume restoration diminishes the threat to the microcirculation by decreasing blood viscosity.

Urinary System

Decreased blood volume causes a decreased blood flow to the kidneys. In addition, burn damage involves damage to blood cells and hemoglobin release, as well as muscle damage, if full-thickness wounds are involved, with myoglobin release. The kidneys are involved in removing the waste from this damage, but the extensive amount of waste could obstruct and damage renal tubules. In addition, the decreased blood flow to the kidneys, if severe, can increase damage to the renal tubules.

> Burn injury → fluid loss and increased blood viscosity with blood and muscle damage → blocked microcirculation and decreased renal perfusion → decreased perfusion of renal cells → ischemia → necrosis → tubular necrosis and decreased renal function → fluid, electrolyte, and acid–base imbalance

Acute tubular necrosis (ATN), ischemia, and death of renal tubules are the greatest threats to the renal system after a burn injury. Tubular necrosis will result in impairment of renal function and fluid and electrolyte, as well as acid–base, imbalances owing to impaired renal function in regulation of these areas.

Respiratory System

Smoke inhalation and damage to respiratory structures owing to heat inhalation can cause bronchiolar constriction and alveolar obstruction or collapse. Additionally, burns to the chest can result in decreased depth of respiration and, if burns are circumferential in the chest area, can restrict breathing severely. Inhalation of carbon monoxide can result in hemoglobin receptors for oxygen being occupied by carbon monoxide, further blocking oxygenation. The ultimate

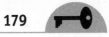

result is decreased ventilation and hypoxia, as well as hypercarbia (high carbon dioxide levels). **4** **5**

> Burn injury → inhalation of smoke and ashes → alveoli blockage → carbon monoxide inhalation → carboxyhemoglobin formation (carbon monoxide binding to oxygen receptors) → heat damage to bronchioles and alveoli → damage and collapse of alveoli → hypoxia and hypercarbia (elevated carbon dioxide) with related imbalances

Related imbalances may include

- Respiratory acidosis owing to increased carbon dioxide levels
- Metabolic acidosis owing to hypoxia, anaerobic metabolism, and lactic acidosis
- Hypochloremia (chloride is excreted as NH_4Cl to buffer acid)
- Hyperkalemia (potassium is shifted out of cells as H^+ ions are shifted into cells to buffer excess acid)
- Hypocalcemia (acidosis causes more calcium to bind with protein, lowering the amount of free Ca^{2+})
- Hyperphosphatemia (more than 4.6 mg/dL [6.6 mg/dL in children] or 1.46 mmol/L [2.2 mmol/L in children] as phosphates move out of the cell and hydrogen ions shift into the cell, although low calcium levels will stimulate excretion of phosphate to prevent the formation of calcium phosphate further decreasing circulating calcium) **4**

Hypercarbia, i.e., elevated carbon dioxide levels, will result in a respiratory acidosis. Respiratory rate may be increased in an attempt to remove carbon dioxide, but blocked airways may make efforts ineffective. Electrolyte shifts to balance acidosis may result.

Additionally, hypoxia results in anaerobic metabolism in tissues with a resulting lactic acidosis. While respirations normally are increased to buffer the metabolic acidosis, damage to the lungs reduces or removes this mechanism from availability. **4** **5**

Treatment for the respiratory damage involves oxygen supplements, intubation, and artificial ventilation when indicated, as well as the use of a hyperbaric chamber to remove carbon monoxide, if needed. Any restriction to the chest owing to burned skin is removed surgically. The nurse must monitor arterial blood gases and oxygen saturation levels to determine the effectiveness of treatment. In addition, the nurse should monitor for signs of acidosis and related acid–base imbalances. **5** **9**

Case Application

Eliza Gentry, age 8, experienced a burn injury to the neck, face, and chest (25 percent of the body with partial- and full-thickness wounds) after a firecracker she was playing with in her room exploded in her face. The room was full of smoke from a resulting fire when Eliza was rescued. While determining how to approach Eliza's care, the nurse considers the following:

Airway: Since oxygen delivery is primary to life, the nurse checks that Eliza's airway is patent and assists the primary-care provider in inserting an endotracheal tube for assistive ventilation. Additional respiratory support likely will include

- Oxygen supplementation
- Suctioning to remove excess secretions and smoke particles
- Hyperbaric chamber if carbon monoxide poisoning is suspected
- Arterial blood-gas determination and oxygen saturation levels to evaluate status

Circulation and urinary systems: Fluid loss is anticipated because significant body surface was affected. Fluid shifts will result in hypovolemia and hemoconcentration. Treatment will include

- Intravenous fluids at a rate calculated for body surface area.
- Albumen infusion as indicated.
- Blood pressure check hourly.
- Urine output (color and amount).
- Intake and output.
- The nurse will closely monitor for signs of renal compromise and related electrolyte and acid–base imbalances.
- Eliza's level of consciousness and orientation will be monitored with the understanding that the causes of alterations could be multiple (e.g., hypovolemia, acidosis, Na^+, Ca^{2+}, and K^+ disturbances). In addition, the nurse will monitor the patient's neuromuscular responses (i.e., Ca^{2+}, K^+, and HPO_4^-). Laboratory values, as ordered, will be monitored for imbalance.

As indicated earlier, patient symptoms may be due to multiple imbalances that occur with injury. It is not essential in all circumstances to determine the precise cause of each symptom. Hypovolemia will be treated and will address circulatory and renal concerns. Treatment of renal symptoms and respiratory difficulties will address electrolyte and acid–base imbalances. If electrolyte imbalance is severe, particularly hypocalcemia, supplementation may be provided. The nurse must monitor for complications of overtreatment with resulting imbalance of the opposite nature (i.e., hypercalcemia). **9**

PREGNANCY

Unlike burn injury, **pregnancy** is a developmental condition that generally progresses along a regular path. It is not a disease or injury to the body but has monumental impact on most systems of the body. Pregnancy also presents the potential for complications owing to the physiologic changes that occur. The "normal" changes that occur in pregnancy that might have an impact on fluid balance and potential acid–base imbalance include **1**

- *Circulatory system*—maternal blood volume rises about 30 percent and cardiac output rises to 30–40 percent above normal until about 27 weeks. The pregnant uterus presses on the large pelvic blood vessels, reducing venous return and causing edema of the feet, along with varicose veins and hemorrhoids.

- *Digestive system*—owing to fetal demand, the mother must consume additional vitamin D to increase calcium absorption; in addition, there is a need for more phosphates.

- *Endocrine and renal systems*
  - Increased production of aldosterone and steroids of pregnancy result in water and sodium retention by the kidneys.
  - The GFR is increased by 50 percent.
  - Urine output is elevated, which allows excretion of metabolic wastes from the fetus and the mother.

- *Respiratory system*
  - Increased need for additional iron (375 mg) for the fetus to avoid anemia, which could affect oxygenation.
  - Minute ventilation increases by 50 percent to meet the 20 percent higher oxygen demands for the fetus and mother's increased metabolic rate and to compensate for shallow breathing as a result of uterine pressure on the diaphragm.
  - Respiratory chemoreceptors have higher sensitivity to CO_2, and increased respiratory rate results in maintenance of P_{CO_2} level lower than normal; thus a slight respiratory alkalosis may be normal during pregnancy.

Thus pregnancy presents a multitude of changes for the expectant mother and places her at risk for several fluid, electrolyte, and acid–base imbalances should any of the body's compensatory mechanisms fail. *Additionally, any preexisting conditions, such as obesity, atherosclerosis, or prediabetes, could convert to fully active conditions.* **1**

The primary complication of pregnancy that places the mother at risk for fluid, electrolyte, and acid–base imbalance in the early stages of pregnancy is hyperemesis gravidarum (prolonged nausea with vomiting). The loss of fluids, decreased intake owing to nausea, and loss of stomach acids predispose the woman to dehydration and alkalosis with related electrolyte imbalance. **8**

The primary complication of pregnancy that places the mother at risk for fluid imbalance is preeclampsia or toxemia of pregnancy. This condition has been associated with abnormal development of the placental artery with thrombosis and maternal organ dysfunction. The primary offending elements in toxemia and symptoms noted are

- Proteinuria.

- Hypertension.

- Facial and upper extremity edema.

- Occurs in third trimester and on occasion in postpartal period.

- May progress to eclampsia and seizures.

- The major treatment is delivery of the baby.

- Fluid volume is managed to avoid hypovolemia and the impact of hypervolemia.

- Treatment also may include infusion of magnesium to decrease the potential for seizure.

- The nurse must monitor closely for signs of hypermagnesemia and for fluid overload or deficit.

- Treatment for high blood pressure could include calcium blockers, which require the nurse to monitor for calcium imbalance.

- Angiotensin-converting enzyme (ACE) inhibitors block angiotensin II to decrease vasoconstriction; this drug also will prevent aldosterone production and sodium and water retention.

As indicated under burn injury, the symptoms manifested by the pregnant patient with fluid, electrolyte, or acid–base imbalances may be multicausal. The nurse must take a thorough history, noting onset and duration of symptoms. The physical assessment is also key. Treatment of the complications associated with pregnancy could result in additional complications if the patient and treatments are not monitored closely. **6**

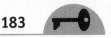

Conclusion

When caring for clients with potential fluid, electrolyte, and acid–base imbalances, the role of the nurse involves consideration of multiple factors that may have an impact. Developmental factors, specifically extreme youth or extreme age, may play a major role in the creation of or recovery from imbalances owing to the immaturity or insufficient organ function as a result of the aging process. Renal conditions in particular play a significant role in fluid, electrolyte, and acid–base balance. Since the renal system removes or retains fluids and electrolytes, as well as acids and bases, in the body, malfunction of this system will have critical results. Burn injury also can have a severe impact on fluid balance owing to fluid shifts and loss of fluids resulting from drainage and evaporation in areas of exposed tissue. The importance of nursing measures to correct fluid imbalances and prevent damage to body systems, such as the renal system, cannot be overemphasized. Additionally, burn injury has the potential to affect the respiratory system if inhalation injury or carbon monoxide is involved. Pregnancy, while not a disease condition, will result in fluid changes owing to the fetal development and support processes. The nurse must be careful to consider all areas of potential concern. Some key points in this chapter include

- Young patients and the elderly may have organ and system insufficiencies that result in fluid, electrolyte, and acid–base imbalances.

- Treatments to address imbalances may require fine-tuning for clients at age extremes. Thus the nurse should monitor patients closely to determine treatment effectiveness or lack thereof.

- Nursing care in patients with renal system disorders must focus on restoring and maintaining adequate volume as well as electrolyte and acid–base balance. Anticipating and preventing renal damage owing to hypovolemia or heart failure owing to fluid overload and electrolyte imbalance are also important priorities for the nurse.

- Clients with burn injury and pregnancy may present with fluid volume concerns. The nurse must provide patient and caregiver education regarding measures needed to maintain fluid and electrolyte balance and detect and report early signs of cardiac or vascular dysfunction so that treatment can be provided promptly.

As stated previously, treatment of fluid and electrolyte imbalance can result in the opposite imbalance, so close monitoring of patient status is important in restoring and maintaining homeostasis.

Final Check-up

1. An 82-year-old malnourished woman has been diagnosed with hypoproteinemia. The nurse should be monitoring the patient for which of the following?

   (a) Heavy breathing

   (b) Bright red spots on the extremeties

   (c) Total-body edema

   (d) Elevated blood pressure

2. Patients of extreme youth and extreme age most commonly share which of the following physiologic risks?

   (a) Dehydration

   (b) Respiratory failure

   (c) Liver spots

   (d) Gastric indigestion

3. The nurse should suspect which of the following in a premature infant with labored breathing?

   (a) Atelectasis

   (b) Hypoxia

   (c) Anaerobic metabolism

   (d) All the above

4. A pregnant woman may present with fluid imbalances secondary to which of the following?

   (a) The gender of the fetus

   (b) Cravings for spicy food

   (c) Difficulty urinating

   (d) Increased fluid volume

5. A patient has been admitted with third-degree burns over 45 percent of his upper body. The primary concern for the attending nurse is to monitor for

   (a) hypovolemia.

   (b) bradycardia.

   (c) pulmonary edema.

   (d) hypertention.

CHAPTER 12

Conditions Resulting in Fluid, Electrolyte, and Acid–Base Imbalances

Learning Objectives

At the end of this chapter, the student will be able to

1. Identify patients at risk for heart failure or endocrine dysfunction.

2. Evaluate selected conditions for risk factors related to fluid imbalance.

3. Evaluate selected conditions for risk factors related to electrolyte imbalance.

4. Evaluate selected conditions for risk factors related to acid–base imbalance.

5. Relate symptoms and assessment data to the identified imbalance(s).

6. Identify diagnostic values associated with imbalances caused by selected conditions.

7. Discuss the potential complications related to treatment of selected conditions.

8. Determine the nursing implications relative to fluid, electrolyte, and acid–base imbalances related to the treatment of selected conditions.

Key Terms

Afterload

Cardiomyopathy

Decompensation

Diabetes insipidus (DI)

Diabetes mellitus

Diabetic ketoacidosis (DKA)

Depolarization

Dysrhythmia

Ejection fraction

Heart failure

Hyperglycemia

Hypoproteinemia

Hyperosmolar hyperglycemic Syndrome (HHS)

Ketonuria

Oncologic conditions

Pancreatitis

Pregnancy

Preload

Pulmonary edema

Syndrome of inappropriate ADH (SIADH)

Heart Failure

Heart failure (HF) is a condition in which the heart is unable to sufficiently propel blood forward from either the right side of the heart to the lungs or the left side of the heart to the systemic circulation and brain. Heart failure can result from any interference in the mechanisms contributing to cardiac output (i.e., the volume of blood exiting the heart). Cardiac output results from the volume with each heartbeat (i.e., stroke volume) times the heart rate. Cardiac output depends on the volume entering the heart (i.e., **preload**) and the pressure against which the heart has to pump (i.e., **afterload**) owing to blood in vessels and constriction of blood vessels. Myocardial contractility, measured as **ejection fraction** (EF—the percentage of

Table 12–1   Defining Characteristics of Systolic and Diastolic Heart Failure

Systolic Failure (Most Common Form)	Diastolic Failure
• Inability of heart to eject blood • Left ventricle is unable to generate adequate pressure for ejection • Reduced ejection fraction (below the normal 55 percent) • Some causes include impaired contractile function (cardiac arrest or **cardiomyopathies**), increased afterload (hypertension), or mechanical abnormalities (valvular heart disease)	• Impaired ability of ventricles to relax and fill during diastole • High filling pressures noted owing to stiff or noncompliant ventricles • Results in pulmonary and systemic venous engorgement • Pulmonary hypertension, pulmonary congestion, ventricular hypertrophy, and a normal ejection fraction • Some causes include left ventricular hypertrophy from prolonged hypertension, aortic stenosis, hypertrophic cardiomyopathy, and possibly myocardial fibrosis (in women)
• Mixed form—weakened muscle and dilated ventricular walls that are unable to relax resulting in poor ejection fraction (< 35 percent), high pulmonary pressures, and biventricular failure	
• All forms of heart failure result in low blood pressure, low cardiac output, and poor renal perfusion.	

total volume filling the ventricles that is ejected with each contraction), and the individual's metabolic state or demands also contribute to cardiac output. Heart failure is identified based on the form of dysfunction noted. The two forms of HF and defining characteristics are identified in Table 12–1. Some individuals will demonstrate a mixed form of HF.

CAUSES

1 The primary contributors to development of HF are coronary artery disease and advancing age. Additional causes include

- Hypertension
- Diabetes
- Obesity
- High serum cholesterol
- Cigarette smoking

HF can be acute or chronic. The acute form of HF occurs as a result of a sudden trauma or assault to the heart, such as occurs in **1**

- Myocardial infarction
- Hypertensive crisis

- Pulmonary embolism
- Thyrotoxicosis
- Ventricular septal defect
- Rupture of papillary muscle (e.g., mitral valve)
- Myocarditis
- **Dysrhythmia** (irregular or abnormal heart Rhythm)

The chronic form of HF develops with a long-standing increase in the workload on the heart that causes the heart muscle to weaken. The common causes of chronic HF include 1

- Coronary artery disease
- Hypertension
- Rheumatic heart disease
- Congenital heart disease
- Cor pulmonale
- **Cardiomyopathy** (weakened heart muscle)
- Anemia
- Bacterial endocarditis
- Valvular disorders

SYMPTOMS

Heart Failure is the most common cause of hospitalization for adults older than 65 years of age. The most common symptoms associated with heart failure are listed below. The complications associated with diminished cardiac output owing to HF account for additional symptoms that may be observed. Symptoms of heart failure include

- Ventricular dysfunction characterized by dysrhythmia and diminished pulse pressure
- Reduced activity tolerance and progressive inability to perform the activities of daily living
- Decreased quality of life with inability to participate in many activities owing to workload on the heart
- Decreased life expectancy unless the heart is replaced, dysrhythmia or increasing loss of heart function with associated decrease in cardiac output and decreased tissue perfusion

Table 12–2   Defining Characteristics of Left-Sided and Right-Sided Heart Failure

Left-Sided Heart Failure	Right-Sided Heart Failure
• Left ventricular heaves • Pulsus alternans (alternating strong and weak pulses) • Tachycardia • S_2 and S_4 heart sounds • Left ventricular hypertrophy (point of maximum impulse [PMI] shifts inferiorly and posteriorly) • Pleural effusion **2** • Crackles/rales (pulmonary edema) • Decreased Pao_2, slightly increased $Paco_2$ (gas exchange) **4**	• Right ventricular heaves • Murmurs • Jugular venous distension • Edema, dependent—anasarca (generalized edema, bilateral extremities, sacral, etc.) • Ascites (abdominal edema) • Hepatomegaly (liver edema) • Weight gain **2** • Tachycardia
• Both right and left ventricular heart failure cause fatigue and a sense of anxiety and depression. Additionally, patients may experience	
Left-Sided Heart Failure	**Right-Sided Heart Failure**
• Dyspnea/shortness of breath, including paroxysmal nocturnal dyspnea (PND) • Shallow respirations (32–40 breaths/min) • Orthopnea (shortness of breath when lying down) • Dry, hacking cough • Nocturia • Frothy pink-tinged sputum (pulmonary edema)	• Right upper quadrant pain • Nausea • Anorexia • GI bloating

HF also can be classified as left-sided and right-sided HF, although total HF will manifest symptoms of biventricular failure (Table 12–2). Left-sided (left ventricular) failure is the most common form of HF. Symptoms result from the blood backup into the left atria and pulmonary veins. The increased pressure causes fluid to leak from the pulmonary capillary bed into the interstitium and then into the alveoli, resulting in **pulmonary edema.** Prolonged left ventricular failure will place pressure on the right side of the heart and cause right-sided HF. Right-sided (right ventricular) HF causes a backup of blood into the right atrium and venous circulation. Venous congestion is manifested in elevated jugular veins and systemic edema. **2**

The manifestations displayed by a patient with HF will vary in severity depending on the patient's current state of health and other chronic illnesses that affect the metabolic demands on the patient. Side effects from some treatments for other conditions could affect the symptoms of HF manifested; for example, a patient taking a pulmonary drug such as theophylline might experience tachycardia, which stresses the heart and causes the heart to fail with accompanying symptoms.

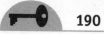
NURSING IMPLICATIONS IN TREATMENT OF HEART FAILURE 6

The treatment for patients in HF centers on the underlying pathology and symptom relief (Table 12–3). Treatment focuses on maintaining a fluid level that the patient's

Table 12–3   Summary of Treatments and Nursing Implications of Heart Failure

Objectives of treatment
1. Decrease intravascular volume—decreases workload on the heart 1
2. Decrease venous return (preload)—decreases workload on the heart
3. Decrease afterload—decreases workload on the heart
4. Improve gas exchange and oxygenation—increases tissue oxygenation in the face of heart failure and decreases perfusion by supplying more oxygen-rich blood
5. Improve cardiac function—strengthens contractions and ejection fraction
6. Reduce anxiety—decreases metabolic demands and decreases workload on the heart

Usual Treatment	Nursing Implications
Treatment of underlying cause will address workload on heart as well as effectiveness of cardiac function depending on cause of heart failure.	Example: If anemia is the cause, iron supplements and patient teaching on nutrition therapy are needed. If thyrotoxicosis is the cause, the patient may undergo thyroid suppression or removal—the nurse monitors for decreased metabolism and complications of hypothyoridism.
High Fowler position	Position decreases venous return while increasing depth of ventilation by lowering diaphragm
Oxygen therapy with pulse oximetry Every hour check blood pressure, heart rate, respiratory rate, intake, and output; continuous ECG 4	Oxygen improves gas exchange and oxygenation Note oxygen values, and monitor respiratory rate, if patient has chronic pulmonary disease; high oxygen levels could suppress breathing Watch closely for dysrhythmia
Cardioversion (atrial fibrillation) Hemodynamic monitoring (cardiac output) Daily weights	Determines effectiveness of treatment on cardiac function; daily weights determine presence of fluid accumulation (1 lb of water = 0.45 kg)
Circulatory assist device, ventricular assist device (VAD), intra-aortic balloon pump → eventual transplantation	Improves cardiac function by regulating contraction; balloon lowers afterload from aortic volume; transplant replaces faulty heart with undamaged heart muscle
Drug therapy • Diuretics—furosemide (Lasix)	Monitor intake and output and monitor for electrolyte imbalance (e.g., sodium and potassium) 7 8
• Nitrates—nitroglycerine	Causes vasodilation, which decreases afterload and thus the workload on the heart
• Inotropics digoxin, dopamine	Strengthen cardiac contractility—watch for signs of return or worsened heart failure owing to increased workload on heart
Nutritional therapy	Dietary approaches to stop hypertension (DASH)
Dietary restriction of sodium—avoid milk, cheese, canned soup or vegetables, bread, cereal	Low (2.5 g) sodium (normal range 7–15 g)

heart can manage while promoting adequate tissue perfusion. Nursing measures will include frequent assessments, interventions, and evaluation of treatment effectiveness.

SPEED BUMP

1. *Which of the following pieces of clinical information indicates that the patient is at risk for heart failure?*
   (a) *Electrocardiogram (ECG) shows a persistent tachycardia.*
   (b) *Blood pressure remains 120 mm Hg systolic.*
   (c) *Urine output is 40 mL/h and yellow.*
   (d) *Cholesterol level is below normal range.*

2. *Which of the following pieces of information in the patient's history would alert the nurse to watch the patient closely for signs of chronic heart failure?*
   (a) *The patient was diagnosed with acute renal failure 1 month ago.*
   (b) *The patient is taking furosemide (Lasix) three times a day.*
   (c) *The patient's hematocrit is consistently below 20 percent.*
   (d) *The patient has a history of controlled asthma.*

Endocrine Conditions: Diabetes Insipidus, Syndrome of Inappropriate ADH (SIADH), and Diabetes (Diabetic Ketoacidosis [DKA] and Hyperosmolar Hyperglycemic Syndrome [HHS])

The integral part that endocrine glands and their hormones play in maintaining fluid and electrolyte balance provides a clear basis why dysfunction in these glands would result in fluid, electrolyte, or acid–base imbalances. Three conditions will be highlighted here to indicate this point.

DIABETES INSIPIDUS

The posterior lobe of the pituitary gland releases antidiuretic hormone (ADH) in response to serum osmolality. High serum osmolality causes the release of ADH, which directs the kidneys to conserve water to restore fluid concentration balance. Low serum osmolality or high blood pressure can result in a neuroendocrine reflex inhibiting the release of ADH, which results in excretion of water and restoration of normal fluid volume and blood pressure, as well as bringing serum osmolality into the normal range. Stretching of the atrial muscle will stimulate the release of atrial natriuretic peptide (ANP), which causes an inhibition of ADH release, resulting in diuresis and a lower fluid volume.

Any condition that inhibits the release of ADH or the renal response to ADH will cause an increase in urinary excretion of water. Injury to the hypothalamus or pituitary gland can inhibit the production or release of ADH. These conditions or any condition blocking renal response to ADH will result in a state of ADH deficiency referred to as **diabetes insipidus (DI).** The main symptom of DI is polyuria. The types and most common causes of DI are

- *Central DI* (i.e., neurogenic)—interference with ADH synthesis or release owing to head trauma, brain tumors, brain surgery, or central nervous system (CNS) infection

- *Neurogenic DI*—inadequate renal response to ADH associated with drug therapy (e.g., lithium), renal damage, or genetic renal disease

A third form of DI that is unrelated to ADH secretion but mimics the polyuria of DI is

- *Psychogenic DI*—excessive water intake resulting from a psychologic disorder or a lesion in the thirst center

The manifestations of DI include

- Polydipsia—intense thirst and consumption of massive fluid volume
- Polyuria—large volumes of urine output
- Elevated serum osmolality
- Hypernatremia
- Nocturia
- Triphasic pattern
  - Acute phase—abrupt onset of polyuria
  - Interphase—urine output moves toward normal
  - Third phase—DI becomes permanent (2 weeks after onset)
- Dehydration
- Weight loss, constipation, poor tissue turgor, hypotension, and tachycardia
- Hypovolemic shock
- CNS manifestations from irritability to coma
- Water-deprivation study results—weight, pulse, urine and plasma osmolality, urine specific gravity, and blood pressure are obtained, and then fluids are

withheld for 8–16 hours with hourly blood pressure and weight checks and urine osmolality tests until findings stabilize or orthostatic hypotension occurs. Then ADH is administered.

- If central DI is present, urine osmolality will rise more than 9 percent.
- If nephrogenic DI is present, no change will be noted.

Treatment and nursing care center on managing fluid and electrolytes and hormone replacement (central DI). Specific measures that may be implemented include

- Central DI
  - Hypotonic saline or dextrose 5% in water (D_5W) titrated to replace urinary output (monitor glucose to avoid hyperglycemic osmotic diuresis)
  - ADH replacement
    - Desmopressin acetate (DDAVP)—watch for weight gain, headache, restless, and signs of hyponatremia and water intoxication as signs of excessive treatment and polyuria with low specific gravity for inadequate dosage. Chronic treatment could result in nasal irritation.
    - Vasopressin (Pitressin, Diapid)
- For partial central DI
  - Chlorpropamide (Diabinese)—potentiates the action of ADH and stimulates exogenous release
  - Carbamazepine (Tegretol)
- Nephrogenic DI
  - Dietary measures (low-sodium diet, e.g., sodium intake of less than 3 g/day
  - Thiazide diuretics—slow glomerular filtration rate → reabsorb more water
    - Hydrochlorothiazide (HydroDiuril)
    - Chlorothiazide (Diuril)
- Sodium intake of less than 3 g/day
- Indomethacin, a nonsteroidal anti-inflammatory agent, to increase responsiveness to ADH (monitor for gastric irritation)
- Monitoring and patient teaching
  - Daily weights
  - Intake and output
  - Urine specific gravity and follow-up laboratory studies needed

The focus in DI treatment is on maintaining adequate hydration in the absence of a key mechanism for fluid retention—ADH. Nursing care includes recognition that excessive therapy could result in fluid overload, as is seen with excessive ADH secretion.

SPEED BUMP

1. *When a patient experiences diuresis secondary to DI, which of the following treatments should the nurse anticipate?*

   (a) *Potassium supplements and intake of fruit such as bananas*

   (b) *A high-phosphate diet with supplements as indicated*

   (c) *Diuretic therapy with drugs such as furosemide (Lasix)*

   (d) *Diet restricting dairy products to reduce intake of calcium*

2. *The nurse would monitor for which of the following signs that the treatment provided to a patient for DI may be excessive?*

   (a) *Jugular venous distension is noted, and breath sounds reveal rales.*

   (b) *The patient has dry mucous membranes and complains of thirst.*

   (c) *The patient demonstrates anxiety and irritability.*

   (d) *The urine output remains at 30 mL/hour for 3 hours.*

SYNDROME OF INAPPROPRIATE ADH (SIADH)

The posterior lobe of the pituitary gland normally releases ADH in response to elevated serum osmolality to direct the kidneys to conserve water and restore fluid concentration balance. A condition referred to as the **syndrome of inappropriate ADH (SIADH),** in which there is an abnormal production or continued secretion of ADH, will result in excessive retention of water regardless of serum osmolality levels. The characteristic symptoms of SIADH are

- Fluid retention

- Serum hypo-osmolality

- Dilutional hyponatremia

- Hypochloremia

- Concentrated urine despite normal or increased intravascular volume

- Normal renal function

Elderly patients have a higher occurrence of SIADH than individuals in other age groups. Additional causes of SIADH include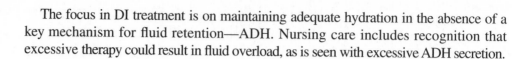

- Malignant tumors
- CNS disorders
  - Head injury—includes skull fracture
  - Brain tumors
  - Infection—encephalitis, meningitis
  - Guillain-Barré syndrome
- Drug therapy
  - Includes opioids, oxytocin, thiazide drugs, antidepressants, and antineoplastics
- Miscellaneous conditions
  - Hypothyroidism
  - Lung infection
  - Chronic obstructive pulmonary disease (COPD)
  - Positive-pressure mechanical ventilation
  - Human immunodeficiency virus (HIV) infection
  - Adrenal insufficiency

Any condition that results in an indiscriminant release of ADH causing retention of fluid and stimulation of thirst will result in SIADH. The specific manifestations of SIADH include **2 3 5**

- Polydipsia—intense thirst and desire to consume massive fluid volumes
- Decreased plasma osmolality
- Low urine output with elevated specific gravity
- Sudden weight gain without edema
- Serum sodium decline—dilutional hyponatremia
  - Muscle cramps and weakness
  - Dyspnea on exertion, fatigue
  - Decreased sensorium
- CNS disorders as sodium levels decline
  - Manifestations from irritability to coma
  - Severe symptoms with Na^+ below 120 mEq/L (120 mmol/L)—possibly related to cerebral edema
    - Anorexia
    - Nausea and vomiting

- Abdominal cramps
- Muscle twitching
- Seizures and coma

Treatment and nursing care center on managing fluid and electrolytes and preventing fluid overload (or deficit). Specific measures that may be implemented include

- Assessment
  - Vital signs, intake and output (all forms)
  - Urine specific gravity
  - Daily weights
  - Level of consciousness
  - Signs of hyponatremia
    - Decreased sensorium
    - Seizures
    - Nausea and vomiting
    - Muscle cramping
  - Heart and lung sounds—signs of fluid overload (heart failure/pulmonary edema)
- Fluid restriction to 1000 mL/day
  - Oral hygiene
  - Distractions to take mind off thirst and fluid restrictions
- Position head of bed flat or at a maximum of 10 degree of elevation to enhance venous return to the heart and increase left atrial filling pressure, reducing ADH release.
- Safety measures to prevent falls owing to altered mental status
- Regular, frequent (every 2 hours) turning, positioning, and range-of-motion exercises if bedridden
- Seizure precautions
- Monitoring and patient teaching
  - Fluid restriction to 800–1000 mL/day
    - Ice chips or sugarless gum to decrease thirst
    - Ration fluid allowance as desired for social occasions
    - Watch for signs and symptoms of fluid overload

- Teach diuretic therapy and side effects ⟨7⟩
  - Potassium and sodium supplements as indicated
  - Dilute supplements to prevent gastric irritation
  - Daily weights (patient teaching on weight process)
  - Monitor intake and output
  - Follow-up laboratory studies needed

The planning and implementation required when caring for a patient with ADH imbalance are similar whether there is a deficit of ADH (DI) or an excess of ADH (SIADH). Fluid concerns are primary and can affect respiratory status (with fluid overload) or circulatory status (with volume deficit or volume overload). A thorough history is required to assist in determining the underlying cause of the condition. Additionally, assistance in the conduct of diagnostic studies, as well as reporting of significant findings from those studies, will aid in early and accurate treatment of the ADH imbalance. In addition to the urinary changes associated with ADH imbalance, neuromuscular and gastrointestinal symptoms are noted with both deficient and excess ADH secretion owing to fluid and electrolyte imbalances. Thus nursing care must address multiple systems and will require interventions and patient teaching from admission past discharge and in some cases through a lifetime of treatment for maintenance of homeostasis. ⟨8⟩

SPEED BUMP

1. *A patient with a head injury is admitted. Which of the following symptoms manifested by the patient is indicative of the development of SIADH?*

   (a) *Complaints of thirst*

   (b) *Dry mucous membranes*

   (c) *Urine output of 400 mL/h*

   (d) *Dyspnea on exertion*

2. *The nurse would monitor for which of the following signs that the treatment provided to a patient with SIADH had been excessive?*

   (a) *The patient has anorexia, nausea, and vomiting.*

   (b) *The patient demonstrates anxiety and irritability.*

   (c) *The urine output remains 30 mL/h for 48 hours.*

   (d) *The patient has an elevated plasma osmolality.*

DIABETIC KETOACIDOSIS (DKA) AND DIABETIC HYPEROSMOLAR SYNDROME OR HYPEROSMOLAR HYPERGLYCEMIC SYNDROME (HHS)

The islets of Langerhans in the pancreas are responsible for producing insulin, the substance required for the metabolism and storage of glucose. Insulin is needed for the transport of glucose across certain cell membranes. The secretion of insulin is stimulated by high glucose, amino acids, and fats and is inhibited by low glucose, amino acid, potassium levels, and high corticosteroid and catecholamine levels. Excess insulin secretion leads to low glucose levels in the blood, stimulating release of glucagon, another hormone released by the pancreas, which increases the production of glucose (gluconeogenesis) from the breakdown of adipose and muscle tissue. This results in the availability of additional glucose and an increased level of glucose in the blood. When adequate insulin is present, glucose is delivered to the tissues for energy, although select tissues can use glucose without the assistance of insulin. If insulin is insufficient or absent or tissues are not responsive to insulin, there is a decreased glucose delivery to the cells.

Diabetes mellitus is a chronic condition related to decreased production or impaired use of insulin or a combination of both. The causes of diabetes mellitus are varied, but the consequence of deficient insulin function is an excessive amount of glucose in the blood (i.e., **hyperglycemia**). There are two types of diabetes mellitus:

- *Type 1*—formerly called *insulin-dependent* or *juvenile diabetes*
  - Occurs commonly before age 30 but can occur at any age
  - Abrupt onset as end result of long-standing assault
  - Less frequent type (5–10 percent of diabetes cases)
  - Minimal or no self-made insulin present
  - Insulin therapy required
  - Nutritional therapy needed
- *Type 2*—formerly called *adult-onset diabetes*
  - Usually occurs after age 35 but can occur at any age
  - Slow, gradual onset; may go undiagnosed for a long period
  - More frequent type (90 percent of diabetes cases)
  - Self-made insulin may be present with minimal tissue responsiveness
  - Insulin therapy may be required for some persons
  - Nutritional therapy is required

Table 12–4   Symptoms of Diabetes Mellitus (Hyperglycemia) and a Complication of Excessive Treatment (Hypoglycemia)

Hyperglycemia	Hypoglycemia
Elevated blood glucose > 126 mg/dL (7.0 mmo/L)	Blood glucose < 70 mg/dL (3.9 mmol/L)
Polyuria (glucose in urine—glycosuria causes an osmotic diuresis)	Cold clammy skin
	Numbness of fingers toes
Polyphagia (increased hunger owing to decreased supply of glucose to cells)	Rapid heart rate (tachycardia)
	Emotional changes
Polydipsia (increased thirst owing to volume depletion from diuresis)	Altered level of consciousness
	Nervousness, tremors
Volume loss → electrolyte imbalance:	Faintness, dizziness
• Headache	Unsteady gait and slurred speech
• Nausea, vomiting, and anorexia	Hunger
• Abdominal cramps	Vision disturbances
• Weakness, fatigue	Seizures → coma
Progressing to severe hyperglycemia	

Regardless of the type of diabetes, two major complications can occur—excess glucose owing to ineffective insulin function and decreased glucose if insulin is provided in excess amounts. The symptoms of diabetes mellitus (hyperglycemia) and a complication of excessive treatment (hypoglycemia) are shown in Table 12–4.

The buildup of glucose presents a distinct problem in fluid, electrolyte, and acid–base balance. One condition that can result for severe hyperglycemia from insufficient insulin or decreased insulin sensitivity is **diabetic ketoacidosis (DKA)**—the buildup of ketones in the blood secondary to the breakdown of fats for energy (because glucose is not available for use). Ketones are metabolic acids that decrease the serum pH, resulting in a metabolic acidosis. In addition, the buildup of ketones will result in **ketonuria,** or loss of ketones in the urine. Along with ketones, electrolytes are lost in the urine, leading to deficits in certain electrolytes. In addition, the high concentration of glucose in the blood will result in an increase in the glucose level in the urine (glucosuria), increasing urine osmolality and resulting in osmotic diuresis with loss of large volumes of fluid. Along with the fluid loss is a loss of electrolytes; thus the patient with ketoacidosis is at risk for dehydration, electrolyte imbalance, and acid–base imbalance. **2 3**

The symptoms that are manifested with DKA result from dehydration secondary to the hyperosmotic state and the resulting fluid and electrolyte imbalance, as well as secondary to the acidosis resulting from use of adipose tissue for energy and the buildup of ketones in the blood. The classic signs of diabetes—polyuria, polydipsia, and polyphagia—are also present.

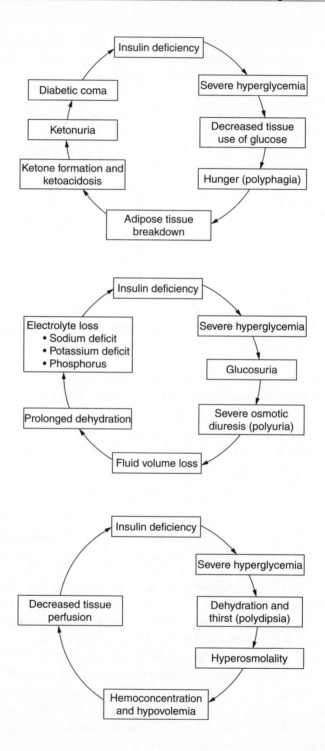

Another condition, less common, that could result from decreased insulin availability or effectiveness also involves the excess buildup of glucose. This condition, referred to as **hyperosmolar hyperglycemic syndrome (HHS),** is an extreme hyperglycemia without the development of ketones. Similar to DKA, HHS results in an osmotic diuresis with loss of fluids in the urine along with a loss of electrolytes. **2   4**

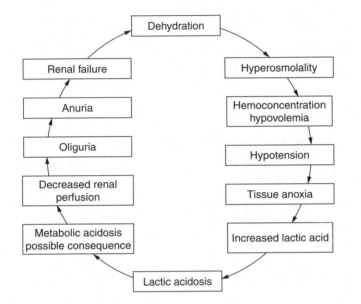

The symptoms of DKA and HHS are similar, with additional symptoms related to the ketone production and buildup. Assessment findings include **3**

- Serum glucose > 300 mg/dL (16.7 mmol/L) in DKA
- Serum glucose > 400 mg/dL (22.25 mmol/L) in HHS
- Thirst (if patient is alert; may be diminished in elderly patients) **5**
- Dry mouth, sunken eyes, flushed dry skin
- Rapid, weak pulse
- Urinary frequency
- Changes in sensorium (from restlessness to confusion to lethargy to coma)
- Glucosuria and ketonuria and fruity (ketone) breath odor (in DKA)
- Deep, rapid breathing (Kussmaul respirations to blow off CO_2)
- Fever (possibly related to dehydration)
- Abdominal pain, nausea, and vomiting

The treatment in both DKA and HHS involves reduction in blood glucose levels through insulin management. Insulin transports glucose into the cells for use. The availability of glucose for energy will stop fat burning for energy and the release of ketones, thus reducing ketoacidosis. Although ketones are not a concern in HHS, reduction of glucose levels remains a critical need. For both DKA and HHS, reduction of blood glucose decreases the osmotic diuresis and decreases loss of water in the urine.

SPEED BUMP

1. *Which of the following symptoms might be noted in a patient with DI or with HHS?*

   (a) *Intense hunger and intake of large meals*

   (b) *High serum potassium levels*

   (c) *Urine output of 300 mL/h*

   (d) *Serum glucose levels above 400 mg/dL*

2. *The nurse would report which of the following pieces of information that would differentiate DI from DKA?*

   (a) *The patient has intense thirst.*

   (b) *The urine output is 400 mL/h.*

   (c) *Serum glucose level is 300 mg/dL.*

   (d) *Potassium level is less than 3.4 mEq/L.*

Conclusion

The role of the nurse when caring for patients with conditions that radically affect the fluid balance of the body and also affect electrolytes and acid–base balance is focused on restoring and maintaining adequate volume as well as electrolyte and acid–base balance. Anticipating and preventing renal damage owing to hypovolemia or heart failure owing to fluid overload and electrolyte imbalance are also important priorities for the nurse. For conditions that are chronic in nature, the nurse must provide patient and caregiver education regarding measures needed to maintain fluid and electrolyte balance and detect and reporting early signs of cardiac or renal dysfunction so that treatment can be provided promptly. As stated previously, treatment of fluid and electrolyte imbalance can result in the opposite imbalance, so close monitoring of patient status is important to restore and maintain homeostasis. **8**

Many conditions, particularly those affecting ADH, can result in imbalances in fluids, electrolytes, and acid–base. Conditions can affect more than one system and result in more than one imbalance. The nurse can anticipate some imbalances based on the specific condition or treatment. Symptoms of the imbalance(s), particularly muscle and nerve dysfunction, including altered level of consciousness, result from fluid, electrolyte, and acid–base imbalance or a combination.

Key points that should be noted from this chapter include

- Heart failure can result from any condition that damages or overstresses the heart and affects preload, afterload, or contractility.
- Right-sided heart failure results in edema of the body and body organs, whereas left-sided heart failure results in edema of the lungs.
- Treatment for heart failure focuses on decreasing volume to decrease preload and afterload and increasing cardiac function, as well as improving cardiac function.
- Treatments must be administered with care to prevent excessive reduction of circulating volume and excessive workload on the heart muscle through drugs that increase cardiac contractions.
- Excessive or deficient ADH can result in an imbalance of fluid, electrolytes, or acid–base.
- Diabetes insipidus (ADH deficiency) results in excessive urinary output and dehydration.
- SIADH (excessive ADH) results in urinary retention and fluid overload.
- Diabetes, insufficient insulin to transport glucose into cells, can result in hyperglycemia and an osmotic diuresis.
- When the body breaks down fats for energy, ketones are produced, resulting in ketoacidosis.
- Osmotic diuresis and ketoacidosis will result in electrolyte shifts and loss and imbalance.
- Symptoms of polydipsia and polyuria are present with conditions that cause diuresis and dehydration.
- Overtreatment of one imbalance could result in the opposite imbalance if care is not exercised.

Case Application

Amisha Pecot, age 23, is admitted with a diagnosis of dehydration. She is groggy but oriented. The vital signs show a blood pressure (BP) of 105/60 mm Hg, a pulse (P) of 126 beats/minute, respiration (R) of 28 breaths/minute, and a temperature (T) of 38°C. Urine output is 15 mL/h of concentrated urine.

The nurse is gathering data to determine the source of the fluid deficit and anticipate treatment and care needed by the patient. What assessments should be made?

- What history assessments would be beneficial to differentiate possible causes of the dehydration? (Ans.: History of previous conditions—diabetes, head injury, cancer, renal disease.)

- What was the patient's previous urine output over the past days (urinary frequency, incontinence, color of urine)?

- What has the patient's fluid intake been over the past days (scant intake or copious intake owing to intense thirst)?

- What other symptoms has the patient had (intense hunger, nocturia, or weight loss)?

Anticipate diagnostic tests that include

- Urinalysis (glycosuria will identify HHS; if ketonuria is present, will indicate DKA); specific gravity will be elevated in each condition—DI, HHS, and DKA.

- Blood glucose (will identify HHS or DKA).

- Water-deprivation study (will determine presence of DI and determine if central DI or nephrogenic DI).

- Electrolytes (indicates the presence of hyponatremia, or if hemoconcentrated, hypernatremia); hypokalemia, venous CO_2, if decreased, indicates acidosis.

Anticipate treatment:

- HHS and DKA—insulin for glucose management, fluid replacement, electrolyte supplement as indicated by laboratory values, with DKA treatment of acidosis if pH is low.

- DI
  - Central DI—ADH replacement or drugs to potentiate action of ADH.
  - Nephrogenic DI—thiazide diuretics.

Question: If a patient is losing fluid owing to lack of the action of ADH, why might a thiazide diuretic be beneficial? (Ans.: Thiazide diuretics slow the GFR and allow for more water reabsorption.)

Monitor results (appropriate treatment will restore fluid and electrolyte and acid–base balance):

- If excessive amounts of ADH are administered, symptoms of SIADH will result.
- If excessive insulin is administered, hypoglycemia will result.
- If excessive fluid replacement is given, fluid overload will result.
- If inadequate or excessive electrolyte therapy is given, electrolyte imbalance will remain.

Appropriate questions and assessments are needed to determine the correct course of treatment and care for a patient. Continued monitoring is necessary to determine if the treatments provided are effective and adequate or insufficient or excessive and to determine the appropriate response.

Final Check-up

1. A 42-year-old patient is admitted after a myocardial infarction. The doctor ordered an intravenous infusion of normal saline at 150 mL/h. Which of the following symptoms would indicate that the patient is experiencing heart failure?

   (a) An increased urine output at 100 mL/h

   (b) A serum potassium level of 4.0 mEq/L (4.0 mmol/L)

   (c) A serum sodium level of 140 mEq/L (140 mmol/L)

   (d) An arterial blood gas indicating a Po_2 of 65 mm Hg

2. The nurse should watch the patient with SIADH who is being treated with fluid restrictions for which of the following signs that the restrictions are effective?

   (a) An arterial blood gas indicating a Po_2 of 85 mm Hg

   (b) A serum sodium level of 133 mEq/L (133 mmol/L)

   (c) A urine output of 25 mL/h of dark yellow urine

   (d) A serum potassium level of 4.0 mEq/L (4.0 mmol/L)

3. Bailey McIntosh is a diabetic with a blood glucose concentration of 320 mg/dL. He has had 300–400 mL of urine each hour over the past 24 hours. The nurse would watch closely for which of the following signs of hemoconcentration and hypernatremia?

   (a) Heavy perspiration

   (b) Diarrhea

(c) Moist mucous membranes

(d) Hyperreflexia

4. The nurse suspects that Mrs. Hung, who has diabetes insipidus, needs desmopressin acetate (DDAVP). Which of the following symptoms would indicate the need for a higher dose of DDAVP?

(a) A sodium level of 125 mEq/L (125 mmol/L) or less

(b) A weight loss of 1 lb or more within 24 hours

(c) Urinary output below 50 mL/h

(d) Polyuria with an elevated serum osmolality

5. Which of the following medication orders would the nurse question for a patient with nephrogenic DI?

(a) Dextrose 5% in water to replace urine output

(b) Desmopressin acetate (DDAVP)

(c) Sodium intake below 3 g daily

(d) Chlorothiazide (Diuril)

References

Needham A. *Comparative and Environmental Physiology Acidosis and Alkalosis.* 2004.

Pagana KD, Pagana TJ. *Mosby's Manual of Diagnostic and Laboratory Tests,* 3rd ed. St. Louis: Mosby Elsevier, 2006.

Saladin K. *Anatomy and Physiology: The Unity of Form and Function,* 4th ed. New York: McGraw-Hill, 2007.

Web Site

http://en.wikipedia.org/wiki/Acidosis

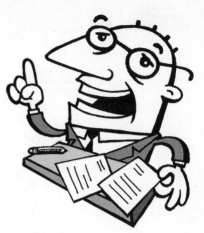

Answers to Final Check-ups

Chapter 1: Key Elements Underlying Fluid and Electrolyte Balance

1. (c) Complaints of thirst
2. (a) High levels of ADH
3. (c) High water retention in extracellular fluid
4. (d) Aldosterone causes potassium loss in the kidneys
5. (b) High calcium levels will cause phosphate to bind with calcium resulting in deposits.

Chapter 2: Key Elements Underlying Acid–Base Balance

1. (d) Acidosis
2. (c) Acidosis

3. (b) Alkalosis

4. (c) Hyperventilation

5. (c) Symptoms of the body's attempt to decrease hydrogen ion retention

Chapter 3: General Nursing Assessments and Diagnostic Tests Related to Fluid, Electrolyte, and Acid–Base Balance

1. (c) Potassium levels of 2.5 mEq/L or lower

2. (a) High levels of sodium owing to hemoconcentration

3. (c) Irritability

4. (a) The patient taking diuretics is at risk for hypokalemia.

5. (d) Numbness and muscle spasm (tetany)

Chapter 4: Fluid Volume Imbalances: Hypovolemia and Hypervolemia

1. (c) The skin is loose and nonelastic.

2. (d) What has Pete had to drink over the last 3 days?

3. (b) Push 50–100 mL of fluids hourly

4. (d) The respiratory rate is increased to compensate for poor circulation.

5. (b) The nurse hears rales in Pete's lung fields.

Chapter 5: Sodium Imbalances: Hyponatremia and Hypernatremia

1. (a) Increased intake of foods such as bananas

2. (b) Aziz Akbar, who is a marathon runner and drinks water for hydration

3. (c) Fluid buildup in extremities and pulmonary edema

4. (c) A past pregnancy resulting in aldosterone deficit

5. (c) Patient's lips and mucous membranes are moist.

Chapter 6: Potassium Imbalances: Hypokalemia and Hyperkalemia

1. (c) Administration of aldactone (spiralactone)

2. (c) Lola Ameriz, who had diarrhea for 3 days

3. (c) Fluid buildup in the extremities and pulmonary edema

4. (a) A report of loose stools six to eight times per day for 4 days

5. (b) Decreased cardiac contractility

6. (a) Patient's heart rate is 70 beats/minute, and rhythm is regular.

7. (c) Has the patient experienced muscle cramps recently?

Chapter 7: Calcium Imbalances: Hypocalcemia and Hypercalcemia

1. (c) 50 percent

2. (c) Polyuria

3. (d) Thiazide diuretic

4. (a) Hyperparathyroidism

5. (d) None of the above

6. (b) A 36-year-old bed-ridden patient who also has lactose intolerance

7. (c) Your hospital stay will be approximately 3 days.

8. (d) Refrain from smoking.

Chapter 8: Magnesium Imbalances: Hypomagnesemia and Hypermagnesemia

1. (c) Administer a magnesium supplement by intramuscular injection.

2. (d) Bob Green, who is homeless and drinks 1 pint of alcohol each day

3. (c) Muscle tremors in the extremities

4. (b) Chronic renal failure and taking Maalox for indigestion

5. (a) The patient's heart rate is 90 beats/minute, and the rhythm is regular.

Chapter 9: Phosphorus Imbalances: Hypophosphatemia and Hyperphosphatemia

1. (a) Thyroid

2. (c) Development of muscle weakness

3. (a) Blood pressure of 170/70 mm Hg

4. (d) Cardiovascular complications.

5. (c) Energy metabolism

6. (b) Frequent reassessment of the patient's knowledge and reteaching

Chapter 10: Acid–Base Imbalances

1. (b) Patient complaints of numbness.

2. (d) A history of prolonged diarrhea

3. (b) Respiratory failure owing to workload on the lungs

Chapter 11: Multisystem Conditions Related to Fluid, Electrolyte, and Acid–Base Imbalances

1. (c) Total-body edema

2. (a) Dehydration

3. (d) All the above

4. (d) Increased fluid volume

5. (a) Hypovolemia.

Chapter 12: Conditions Resulting in Fluid, Electrolyre, and Acid–Base Imbalances

1. (d) An arterial blood gas indicating a Po_2 of 65 mm Hg

2. (d) A serum potassium level of 4.0 mEq/L (4.0 mmol/L)

3. (d) Hyperreflexia

4. (d) Polyuria with an elevated serum osmolality

5. (b) Desmopressin acetate (DDAVP)

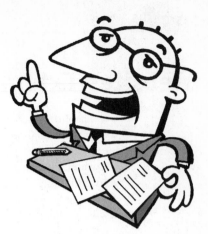

References

Johnson JY. *Handbook for Brunner & Suddarth's Texbook of Medical Surgical Nursing,* 11th edition. Philadelphia: Lippincott Williams & Wilkins, 2008.

Metheny NM. *Fluid and Electrolyte Balance: Nursing Considerations*, 4th ed. Philadelphia: Lippincott Williams & Wilkins, 2000.

Needham A. *Comparative and Environmental Physiology: Acidosis and Alkalosis.* 2004.

Pagana KD, Pagana TJ. *Mosby's Manual of Diagnostic and Laboratory Tests*, 3rd ed. St. Louis: Mosby Elsevier, 2006.

Saladin KS. *Anatomy and Physiology: The Unity of Form and Function*, 4th ed. New York: McGraw-Hill, 2007.

Seely R, Stephens TD, Tate PO. *Anatomy and Physiology*, 7th ed. New York: McGraw-Hill, 2007.

Smeltzer S, Bare B, Hinkle J, Cheever K. *Brunner & Suddarth's Texbook of Medical Surgical Nursing,* 11th ed. Philadelphia: Lippincott Williams & Wilkins, 2008.

Wilson BA, Shannon MT, Shields KM, Stang CL. *Prentice-Hall Nurses' Drug Guide 2008.* Englewood Cliffs, NJ: Prentice-Hall, 2008.

Websites/External Links

www.nephrologychannel.com/electrolytes/hypokalemia.shtml

www.ccmtutorials.com/misc/phosphate/page_05.htm

http://labtestsonline.org/understanding/analytes/phosphorus/test.html

www.nlm.nih.gov/medlineplus/ency/article/000307.htm

www.nlm.nih.gov/medlineplus/druginfo/natural/patient-phosphorus.html

www.emedicine.com/emerg/topic266.htm

www.emedicine.com/emerg/topic278.htm

www.emedicine.com/med/topic1135.htm

www.hoptechno.com/book29o.htm

www.cc.nih.gov/ccc/patient_education/procdiag/24hr.pdf

www.meb.uni-bonn.de/cancer.gov/CDR0000062737.html

www.clevelandclinicmeded.com/dieasemanagement/endocrinology/hcalcemia/hcalc.

www.healthsystem.virginia.edu/uvahealth/peds_hrnewborn/hypocal.cfm

www.healthatoz.com/healthatoz/Atoz/common/standard/transform.jsp?requestURI=/h.

www.emedicine.com/emerg/topic271.htm

www.emedicine.com/emerg/topic1097.htm

www.emedicine.com/emerg/topic1135.htm

www.ecureme.com/emyhealth/data/Hypophosphatemia.asp

www.bookrags.com/Hyperphosphatemia

www.chemocare.com/MANAGING/hyperphosphatemia_hypophosphatemia.asp

www.jfponline.com/Pages.asp?AID=1871&UID

www.euremem.com/emyhealth/data/Hypomagnesemia.asp

http://en.wikipedia.org/wiki/Acidosis

http://en.wikipedia.org/wiki/Hypophosphatemia

http://en.wikipedia.org/wiki/Phosphorus

INDEX

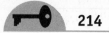

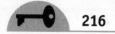

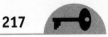

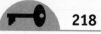

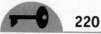

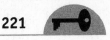

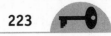

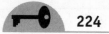

ARF manifestation in/treatment of, 173t

elderly v. complications associated with, 164–165

neural mechanisms, fluid volume regulated by, 9–10

normovolemic hypotonic hyponatremia, 88

nursing assessments

BUN imbalance v., 54

calcium imbalance v., 49–51

chloride imbalance v., 48–49

creatinine imbalance v., 54

electrolyte imbalance v., 43–54

fluid balance v., 33

fluid/electrolyte/acid-base balance, 30–56

magnesium imbalance v., 51–52

phosphate imbalance v., 52–53

potassium imbalance v., 43–46

sodium imbalance v., 46–48, 82–83

terms relating to, 30b

urine, 33

O

oliguria, 170

oncotic pressure

hydrostatic pressure v., 64–65, 65f

solutes in fluid exerting, 9

Osm. *See* osmoles

osmolality, 6

fluid regulation depending on, 9

Na^+ in extracellular, 80

serum, 32–33

urine, 33

osmoles (Osm), 31

electrolytes measured using, 31

osmosis, 5, 8

osmotic pressure, hydrostatic pressure v., 9, 9f

osteomalacia, as hypocalcemia symptom, 114, 120b

osteopenia, 164

osteoporosis

as hypocalcemia symptom, 114, 120b

magnesium preventing, 124

in multisystem conditions, 164

oxalic acids, calcium absorption/hypocalcemia v., 113, 116b

P

parathyroid gland

in calcium regulation, 114

in neonatal hypocalcemia, 113

removal v. hypercalcemia, 119

parathyroid hormone (PTH)

absorption/metabolism v. magnesium, 125

in calcium regulation, 114

hypocalcemia tests v., 114, 115b

phosphate levels v., 138

pH, 20–21

blood, 148

chemical buffer system v., 25

renal system control of, 24–25

respiratory control of, 23–24

pH balance. *See* acid-base balance

phosphate (HPO_4^-)

absorption increased by vitamin D, 137

acid-base balance v., 137

ATP bonds provided by, 136

in cell structure/blood cells, 137

Crohn disease v. absorption of, 140

in electrolyte balance, 12t, 14

electrolytes influencing levels of, 138

in energy metabolism, 137

factors elevating levels of, 142–143

in foods, 141, 141b

imbalance v. nursing assessment, 52–53

influences on cellular uptake of, 138

levels in adults/children/infants, 139

medications v. absorption of, 138

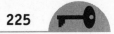

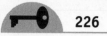

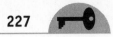